Stop and rest for a minute. Then try again, with the opposite arm raised this time. Again, record your observations.

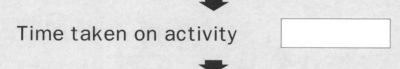

Suggested timings are given for each activity. These are only a guide. You may like to note how long it took you to complete this activity, as it may help in planning the time needed for working through the sessions.

Time taken on activity

Time management is important. While we recognise that people learn at different speeds, this pack is designed to take 20 study hours (your tutor will also advise you). You should allocate time during each week for study.

Take some time now to identify likely periods that you can set aside for study during the week.

	Mon	Tues	Wed	Thurs	Fri	Sat	Sun
am							
pm							
eve							

At the end of the learning pack, there is a learning review to help you assess whether you have achieved the learning objectives.

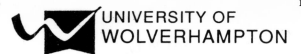
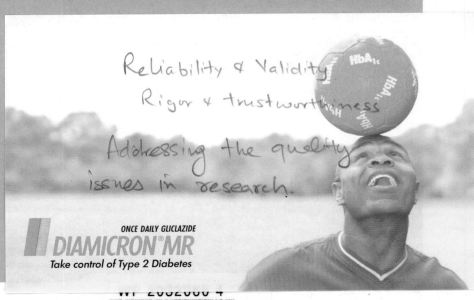

Reliability & Validity
Rigor & trustworthiness

Addressing the quality
issues in research.

ONCE DAILY GLICLAZIDE
DIAMICRON®MR
Take control of Type 2 Diabetes

USING THIS WORKBOOK

The workbook is divided into 'Sessions', covering specific subjects.

In the introduction to each learning pack there is a learner profile to help you assess your current knowledge of the subjects covered in each session.

Each session has clear learning objectives. They indicate what you will be able to achieve or learn by completing that session.

Each session has a summary to remind you of the key points of the subjects covered.

Each session contains text, diagrams and learning activities that relate to the stated objectives.

It is important to complete each activity, making your own notes and writing in answers in the space provided. Remember this is your own workbook—you are allowed to write on it.

Now try an example activity.

ACTIVITY

This activity shows you what happens when cells work without oxygen. This really is a physical activity, so please only try it if you are fully fit.

First, raise one arm straight up in the air above your head, and let the other hand rest by your side. Clench both fists tightly, and then open out your fingers wide. Repeat this at the rate of once or twice a second. Try to keep clenching both fists at the same rate. Keep going for about five minutes, and record what you observe.

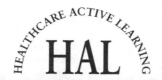

HEALTHCARE ACTIVE LEARNING

HAL

QUALITATIVE RESEARCH METHODOLOGY

in nursing and healthcare

Collette Clifford PhD MSc DANS DipN RGN OND RNT

Reader in Health and Nursing Studies
School of Health Sciences
University of Wolverhampton

THE OPEN LEARNING FOUNDATION

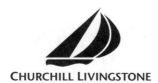

CHURCHILL LIVINGSTONE

NEW YORK EDINBURGH LONDON MADRID MELBOURNE SAN FRANCISCO AND TOKYO 1997

CHURCHILL LIVINGSTONE
Medical Division of Longman Group UK Limited

Distributed in the United States of America by Churchill
Livingstone Inc., 650 Avenue of the Americas, New York,
N.Y. 10011, and by associated companies, branches and
representatives throughout the world.

First published 1997

ISBN 0 443 05738 9

British Library of Cataloguing in Publication Data
A catalogue record for this book is available from the
British Library.

Library of Congress Cataloging in Publication Data
A catalogue record for this book is available from the
Library of Congress

Produced through Longman Malaysia, PP

For The Open Learning Foundation

Director of Programmes: Leslie Mapp
Series Editor: Peter Birchenall
Programmes Manager: Kathleen Farren
Production Manager: Steve Moulds

For Churchill Livingstone

Director (Nursing and Allied Health): Peter Shepherd
Project Controller: Derek Robertson
Project Manager: Valerie Burgess
Design Direction: Judith Wright
Sales Promotion Executive: Maria O'Conner

CONTENTS

	Page
Introduction	1
Learning Profile	2
Session One: Qualitative research design–some background issues	5
Session Two: Approaches to qualitative design	19
Session Three: Collecting data in qualitative design	39
Session Four: Analysing qualitative data	59
Session Five: Reading and using qualitative design research reports	77
Session Six: Writing a research proposal for qualitative design	87
Learning Review	97
Resources Section	99
1 The strengths and weaknesses of quantitative and qualitative research: what method for nursing?	100
2 The psychosocial needs of patients who have attempted suicide by overdose	106
References	115
Glossary	117

OPEN LEARNING FOUNDATION
TEAM MEMBERS

Writer: Collette Clifford,
Reader in Health and Nursing Studies,
School of Health Sciences,
University of Wolverhampton

Editor: Pip Hardy

Reviewers: Dr A. Seed
University of Huddersfield

Dr M. Johnson,
University of Manchester

Series Editor: Peter Birchenall
OLF Programme Head,
Health and Nursing,
University of Humberside

THE OPEN LEARNING FOUNDATION

Higher education has grown considerably in recent years. As well as catering for more students, universities are facing the challenge of providing for an increasingly diverse student population. Students have a wider range of backgrounds and previous educational qualifications. There are greater numbers of mature students. There is a greater need for part-time courses and continuing education and professional development programmes.

The Open Learning Foundation helps over 20 member institutions meet this growing and diverse demand – through the production of high-quality teaching and learning materials, within a strategy of creating a framework for more flexible learning. It offers member institutions the capability to increase their range of teaching options and to cover subjects in greater breadth and depth.

It does not enrol its own students. Rather, The Open Learning Foundation, by developing and promoting the greater use of open and distance learning, enables universities and others in higher education to make study more accessible and cost-effective for individual students and for business through offering more choice and more flexible courses.

Formed in 1990, the Foundation's policy objectives are to:

- improve the quality of higher education and training

- increase the quantity of higher education and training

- raise the efficiency of higher education and training delivery.

In working to meet these objectives, The Open Learning Foundation develops new teaching and learning materials, encourages and facilitates more and better staff development, and promotes greater responsiveness to change within higher education institutions. The Foundation works in partnership with its members and other higher education bodies to develop new approaches to teaching and learning.

In developing new teaching and learning materials, the Foundation has:

- a track record of offering customers a swift and flexible response

- a national network of members able to provide local support and guidance

- the ability to draw on significant national expertise in producing and delivering open learning

- complete freedom to seek out the best writers, materials and resources to secure development.

Other titles in this series

Experimental Research 1 - An introduction to experimental design

Experimental Research 2 - Conducting and reporting experimental research

Research Methodology in Nursing and Healthcare

Evaluative Research Methodology in Nursing and Healthcare

Inferential Statistics in Nursing and Healthcare

Descriptive Statistics

INTRODUCTION

This unit is designed to give a broad introduction to qualitative research design. We will be exploring different approaches to qualitative research, including ethnography, phenomenology and grounded theory. We will also be considering ways in which a researcher undertaking qualitative research collects and analyses data using observation and interviewing techniques. We hope that on completion of the unit you will be able to:

- distinguish between qualitative and quantitative methodology

- define research problems that lend themselves to qualitative approaches

- critically read nursing and health research journals and articles employing qualitative methodology

- design a small-scale research study using qualitative methodology.

Each unit is estimated to take 20 hours of study. Within each session there are a number of activities designed to help your learning and these also have suggested times. However, you should be aware that the time allocated is only an estimate – some people may take longer than others in different activities. It does not matter if it takes you more or less than the suggested time to complete each activity as long as you understand the principles explored at the end of it.

Session One is designed to help you understand the processes involved in qualitative research design which we are to discuss in more depth in subsequent sessions. To develop a clear understanding of this topic we will initially explore the way knowledge is developed and then consider the distinction between inductive and deductive reasoning.

Session Two introduces a range of different approaches to qualitative research design and considers how these can be used. We begin by exploring how qualitative research design differs from quantitative research design and then consider the basic ideas of using qualitative design for the purpose of exploration and description.

Session Three considers data collection in qualitative design. We begin by exploring when it is appropriate to use interview techniques to collect data and continue by looking at the stages involved in collecting data via interviews. The strengths and weaknesses of the interview approach will be discussed. We then examine when it is appropriate to use observation techniques to collect data. Finally, we consider how data can be collected through observation and discuss the strengths and weaknesses of the observation approach.

Session Four considers ways in which we might analyse qualitative data. We explore 'content analysis' and use worked examples to help you understand this process.

Session Five explores the key points you need to consider to help you critically read and understand published qualitative research. This should help identify situations in which qualitative research can be used in practice.

Session Six focuses on writing for qualitative design. The purpose of this is to help plan a research study using a qualitative approach and to write a research proposal for it.

Learning Profile

Given below is a list of learning outcomes for each session in this unit. You can use it to identify your current learning and to consider how the unit can help you to develop your knowledge and understanding. The list is not intended to cover all the aspects discussed in every session and so the learning profile should be used only for general guidance.

For each of the learning outcomes listed below tick the box that corresponds most closely to the point you feel you are at now. This will provide you with an assessment of your current understanding and confidence in the areas you will study in the unit.

	Not at all	Partly	Quite well	Very well

Session One

I can:

- identify the influences which shape our views of the world ☐ ☐ ☐ ☐
- distinguish between inductive and deductive reasoning in research ☐ ☐ ☐ ☐
- explain how inductive and deductive reasoning influence theory development. ☐ ☐ ☐ ☐

Session Two

I can:

- describe the basic principles of qualitative design ☐ ☐ ☐ ☐
- discuss a range of different approaches to qualitative research design ☐ ☐ ☐ ☐
- match research questions to an appropriate research design ☐ ☐ ☐ ☐
- explain what is meant by the term 'triangulation' ☐ ☐ ☐ ☐
- discuss the concepts of validity and reliability in the context of qualitative research ☐ ☐ ☐ ☐
- outline the potential ethical dilemmas researchers may face when completing qualitative research studies. ☐ ☐ ☐ ☐

Session Three

I can:

- identify when it is appropriate to use interview techniques to collect data ☐ ☐ ☐ ☐
- explain the stages involved in collecting data via interviews ☐ ☐ ☐ ☐

	Not at all	Partly	Quite well	Very well

Session Three *continued*

- discuss the strengths and weaknesses of the interview approach □ □ □ □
- establish when it is appropriate to use observation techniques to collect data □ □ □ □
- outline how data can be collected through observation □ □ □ □
- describe the strengths and weaknesses of the observational approach. □ □ □ □

Session Four

I can:

- describe how data collected in qualitative studies can be broken down into data display, reduction and interpretation □ □ □ □
- explain how to undertake content analysis □ □ □ □
- report findings from qualitative research □ □ □ □
- recognise how to analyse data in different approaches to qualitative research. □ □ □ □

Session Five

I can:

- critically read a published research study that has used qualitative research design □ □ □ □
- distinguish between research reports that have a descriptive/exploratory orientation and those which have an interpretative orientation of ethnography, phenomenology and grounded theory □ □ □ □
- discuss how qualitative research can be used to influence practice and further development of knowledge. □ □ □ □

Session Six

I can:

- plan a research study using a qualitative approach □ □ □ □
- write a research proposal for qualitative design. □ □ □ □

Qualitative research design – some background issues

Introduction

The purpose of this session is to introduce you to the subject of qualitative research design. The information in it is designed to help you understand the processes involved in qualitative research design which we will be looking at in more depth in subsequent sessions. When we use the term 'qualitative research' we are using a broad term to describe a variety of different approaches to research. Although these approaches differ, there are common features in the way the research is approached.

In order to develop a clear understanding of the topic we will begin by exploring how knowledge is developed. We will then consider the distinction between inductive and deductive reasoning – the ways in which we think about the world around us.

Session objectives

When you have completed this session you should be able to:

- identify the influences which shape our views of the world
- distinguish between inductive and deductive reasoning in research
- explain how inductive and deductive reasoning influence theory development
- describe how researchers gather information.

1: Finding out about the world

To begin our explanation of qualitative research we need to think about how it is we find out about the world around us.

Every day we are surrounded by many different sources of information. We talk to people and watch how they behave in every-day life, we read newspapers and books, we watch television and listen to the radio, we might use the Internet. All of these sources of information help to shape our perception and form our opinions of the world around us. As a result of these experiences we make judgements about situations we observe and make plans for our own activities. We even attempt to shape other people's views by expounding our own 'theories of life'.

Whilst all this is a perfectly normal response to every-day existence, there are times, for example when we are conducting research, when we need to be able to distinguish between our own personal views, based on our experiences, and a more objective assessment of a situation.

ACTIVITY 1 — ALLOW 10 MINUTES

Look at the following list of potential sources of information and try to put them into the following categories.

1   Authority figures.

2   Interpretative material.

3   Factual information.

4   Personal experience.

- parents/family
- teachers
- friends/peer group
- managers/mentors/colleagues at work
- factual books (text books)
- novels
- newspapers
- popular magazines
- professional/academic journals
- television – entertainment
- television – documentary
- radio – entertainment
- radio – documentary
- theatre
- films
- using the Internet
- observing the world
- listening to others around you
- intuition.

Commentary

Group 1: Authority figures	Group 2: Interpretative material	Group 3: Factual information	Group 4: Personal experience
● parents/family	● novels	● factual books (text books)	● observing the world
● teachers	● popular magazines	● professional/ academic journals	● listening to others around you
● friends/peer group	● television – entertainment	● television – documentary	● intuition
● managers / mentors	● radio – entertainment	● radio – documentary	
	● theatre	● newspapers	
	● films	● using computers/ Internet	

Table 1: Categorisation of sources of information.

Types of knowledge

Categorisation helps us to consider the *nature* of the knowledge gained from all of these different sources. The questions we need to ask here are:

- how reliable is this knowledge?

- how exactly has this knowledge shaped my views of the world?

Authority figures

In Group 1 in *Table 1* we have listed the *people* who might influence your attitudes and views in life. It is well known that parental influence is a very potent form of learning and shaping our knowledge about the world around us. You only have to watch how children mimic their parents' actions to see this. As we grow older we also learn from our teachers in school and college. Eventually, when we go to work we learn from our 'teachers' at work – our colleagues and those people who manage us or act as mentors. We may believe that what our parents and teachers tell us is 'true' because they are the figures of *authority* in our lives and as such seem reliable sources of information.

ACTIVITY 2
ALLOW A FEW MINS

Think about the authority figures you have known in you life and the ways they influenced your outlook on life.

Commentary

Here are a few of our own responses.

- my parents led me to believe it is best not to take risks

- my school teachers emphasised that success in school would enable me to have a better choice of career

- my old boss made me feel that success in my work was related to the number of hours I worked.

Interpretative statements

In Group 2 in *Table 1* we have included a range of material such as books and plays that can be loosely classed as offering *interpretations* of the world. Most entertainment of the kind listed offers us ways of looking at the world through the eyes of someone else. Other people's interpretations of the world help shape our personal view of the world. These experiences may reinforce our existing views (such as those our parents gave us), but by debating and discussing our reactions to books and films, for example, we further refine our world view.

| ACTIVITY 3 | ALLOW 2 MINUTES |

Think about the books, plays or television programmes that have influenced you. How strong was this influence?

Commentary

We will, obviously, have had different experiences and have reacted differently to them. It is not unusual for a film, television programme or book to change our way of looking at the world. For example, a successful television series of life in earlier centuries, such as the screening of novels by Charles Dickens or Jane Austen, can cause us to consider the complexity of social life and relationships in our own century in a new light.

Factual information

In Group 3 of *Table 1* we have listed sources of information that present a more objective view of the world. For example, television and radio documentaries, text books and professional and academic journals and newspapers would claim to present simply the 'facts'. The challenge, however, is to draw out what actually constitutes 'facts' and to distinguish these from personal viewpoints or individual interpretations of the world.

ACTIVITY 4 · ALLOW 60 MINUTES

Try to watch or listen to a television or radio documentary programme in an area you already know something about, or that interests you, and then consider the following points.

1   How much factual information was presented in terms of the percentage of time spent on facts?

2   Where did the facts come from? Were they one person's experience and views or were they representative of a larger group of people?

3   Did the presentation concentrate solely on the facts or was it in any way an interpretation of the facts?

4   Given your own knowledge of the subject, were any areas omitted? (selective reporting)

Commentary

We cannot comment on the particular programme you watched or listened to but this activity should serve to make you think a little more about how knowledge can be presented. You might have watched a programme discussing euthanasia in which a group of people participated who were strongly orientated towards euthanasia. The choice of such a group might have been influenced by the programme producer's own views of euthanasia. This should serve to demonstrate that a constant questioning of facts and seeking out of bias is important in research.

Personal experience

In Group 4 of *Table 1* we have put observations and lessons we learn from the world around us as a result of our own *personal experience*. As our experience develops we begin to challenge the authority of the people identified in Group 1 and through discussion with our friends and peers to look beyond what this influential group has to say. Life itself begins to shape our opinions. For example, you might have been told by your parents that hard work will bring success in your job. You might, however, learn by experience that hard work *isn't* enough and that you also need to be good at dealing with office politics. It is the combination of knowledge sources with our own experience that gives us our own personal view of the world.

All four of these ways of acquiring knowledge can be used in developing research studies. For example, the literature review conducted in the course of a research study may include drawing on existing texts and opinions and examining what 'authorities' say on a given subject. In the same way facts can be drawn from the literature. Researchers use this information in combination with their own reasoning, drawn from their own experiences.

The personal interpretation the researcher uses will draw on various forms of reasoning. We now need to consider in more detail the reasoning processes we might use in developing knowledge in relation to research.

2: Inductive and deductive reasoning

To understand the principles of qualitative research design we need to consider not only the sources of knowledge but also the ways in which we *develop* that knowledge. Broadly speaking, there are two approaches to developing knowledge – 'inductive' and 'deductive' reasoning.

Inductive reasoning: using observation to formulate an idea or theory.

Inductive reasoning can be described very simply as the first step in knowledge development. This is the process by which we unearth knowledge and identify facts. In observing a situation of which little is known we may be able to *bring knowledge into view*. Alternatively, sometimes we can look again at some established facts and discover that maybe we have taken too much for granted and that such 'facts' can be challenged.

Deductive reasoning: taking a known idea or theory and applying it to a situation.

Deductive reasoning can be seen as a second step in the process of developing knowledge. Using the deductive approach we might take some aspect of *knowledge that has previously been identified* and apply that to a new situation.

We will now consider each of these in more detail.

Inductive reasoning

To explore what we mean by saying that inductive reasoning is the first step in developing knowledge let us imagine the situation faced by the early medical scientist Harvey in the sixteenth century. Harvey, who is credited with discovering how the circulation of the blood works, knew little about how the body worked. He had no text books to outline the facts about how the various body systems work. Harvey probably went through a process of inductive reasoning to make his discovery. The idea that blood circulation is controlled by the pumping action of the heart was gradually discovered by connecting a number of ideas. It is likely that Harvey observed the external features of the circulation, such as skin colour. This can be seen as the inductive phase of this process of knowledge development. He might then have suggested a relationship between skin colour and the circulation of the blood. In this way inductive reasoning was used to bring knowledge into view, by observing situations and making links between such observations.

Another example of inductive reasoning can be found in the work of the early psychological theorist Piaget. Piaget observed his own children at different stages of development and, on the basis of these observations, *concluded* that skill development in children occurs at different ages and so proposed a *theory* of development.

In day-to-day life we follow very similar processes to those of Harvey and Piaget. We make observations, perhaps of the way people react in certain situations, and develop conclusions (make inferences) about the world around us on this basis.

ACTIVITY 5   ALLOW 5 MINUTES

List three situations in your life where you may have used inductive reasoning.

1

2

3

Commentary

You are probably unconsciously applying an inductive reasoning approach to your thinking in a lot of every-day situations. For example, when you start a new college programme or a new job you probably know the basic principles about the course you are going to undertake or the work that you are about to do, but there will be aspects of doing that course or job that are not so easy to define. These might include:

● understanding how your peer group work together

● understanding how people in that organisation work together

● knowing what other people think or feel about their work.

As a result of your subsequent experiences you might formulate some ideas about how the organisation works. You will have observed what is going on around you and put your own interpretation on the situation. From your *observations* you make some *inferences* about the situation.

Deductive reasoning

Deductive reasoning involves drawing from ideas or theories that have already been established in one context and making conclusions about them in another context.

Let's return to our example about the circulation of the blood. Harvey spent some time pondering about how the body worked and, through a process of induction, identified certain features of the circulation. With a good working knowledge of how water pumps work, he took that knowledge and proposed that the circulation of the blood worked in the same way. In thinking about the heart as a pump he could *apply* existing knowledge about pumping to the circulation of the blood and could have proposed that when the heart beats faster then blood will circulate faster around the body. In this way, Harvey used deductive reasoning, applying existing principles to a new situation.

ACTIVITY 6 — ALLOW 5 MINUTES

List three situations in your life where you might use deductive reasoning.

1

2

3

Commentary

You will probably have thought of a number of situations in which you do this. In your professional work you are probably using this process every day – applying established ideas or theories to your own practices. If you are working with people you may have a lot of ideas or theories about how people function which influence your work. You may, for example, know about theories of bereavement and be able to use them with people who have experienced some other kind of loss. You might deduce that people who lose their health or the use of a limb may well go through the same stages of grief as someone who loses their husband or wife.

ACTIVITY 7 — ALLOW 5 MINUTES

Review the following situations and state whether they are examples of inductive or deductive reasoning.

1 A group of people on holiday in the Mediterranean decide that they will not lie in the sun as this may increase the risk of skin cancer occurring.

2 A man travelling to work misses the train at 8.15 am but decides he will wait on the station for the next train which he assumes will arrive in the next 15 minutes.

3   A care assistant working in a nursing home notes that over several meals a lot of food has been left by the residents. She infers that this is indicative of some problem and decides to investigate further by asking the residents what they feel about the food.

4   When travelling to college a student starts to talk to some homeless people. In the course of the conversation several of the homeless people indicate that they did not want to leave their homes but that their circumstances had forced them to. The student changes her views about the causes of homelessness as she had previously assumed most people were homeless by choice.

Commentary

1   This is an example of deductive reasoning. The group of people on holiday have heard the facts associated with skin cancer and exposure to the sun and decided to use that knowledge in their own situation.

2   The man in this situation feels quite confident about waiting for the next train because his *previous experience* has told him that if he misses one train another will arrive. Again, this is a process of deductive reasoning based on knowledge of train frequency and times.

3   This is an example of inductive reasoning. The care assistant has made some *observations* that suggest there may be a problem. She has *inferred* from the data presented that it may be due to the quality of the food.

4   Again, this is an example of inductive reasoning. The student had an *idea* about homelessness that was challenged when she began to listen to the perspective of the homeless people. From this perspective she *inferred* there were other causes of homelessness than that she had previously identified.

3: Using inductive and deductive reasoning in research

The reason it is important to know how knowledge is developed and about the reasoning processes involved is because this is linked very closely with the way in which researchers develop theory. In this context a **theory** is a *perception of reality in which concepts are identified, relationships proposed and the results arising out of those relationships predicted*. This might seem quite a complex statement, so we will now consider it in a little more detail.

Theory development

The first step in theory development is *identifying the concepts* relating to a particular situation. If we consider unemployment for example, you might have observed certain characteristics of people you know who are unemployed. You might have noted that these people appear to be depressed, have little energy and suffer from lack of motivation to get involved in other aspects of life. If you did

Theoretical sampling: *an approach used in sampling in grounded theory in which the sampling technique is based on the concepts that have theoretical relevance to the evolving theory.*

notice this what you have done is to identify certain 'concepts' or factors relating to being unemployed by using a process of inductive reasoning.

Once the concepts have been identified then it is possible to propose relationships between them. This is the second step in theory development. So, for example, you might propose that there is a link between the concept of unemployment and the concept of depression. What you are doing here is beginning to formulate a theory – that is, you are *stating a relationship between two concepts* (unemployment and depression) and suggesting that there may be a link. (In research such concepts are described as **variables**).

Variable: the term used to describe the characteristics or features of the objects or people in a research study.

You would not be able to propose such a link *unless the concepts had been identified in the first place*. This is the broad distinction between inductive and deductive reasoning and it is a principle which is reflected in qualitative and quantitative research approaches. Inductive reasoning works at the level of concept identification, unearthing the ideas as a basis for development. Once a relationship between concepts has been proposed then a basis for testing the theory has been established. Once the concepts have been established we start to move into the realms of deductive reasoning, for we are beginning to work with 'known' ideas. If, following the proposed testing, it is found that the relationship does exist, then the proposed theory can be accepted as true.

Let us consider a situation in which we observe a group of students undertaking a programme at a local college. In our discussions with these students we find that they do not answer our questions as quickly as might be expected and we eventually infer from our observations that the students lack energy and appear to be excessively tired. We would then ask 'why is this?' We might give several reasons for this phenomenon, such as excessive work or excessive partying and we might extend our enquiries to identify which of these factors appear to be associated with this situation. In so doing we might find that the student who appeared to be the most tired had the heaviest workload in their college programme. Consequently we might propose a relationship between the students' energy level and the volume of work they had to do. Whilst we can suggest that this relationship exists we cannot confidently state that it does unless we undertake some further research. In this situation we have gone through a process of identifying concepts – tiredness and workload – proposed a relationship between them and are now ready to test this hypothesis through research. *Figure 1* illustrates this process.

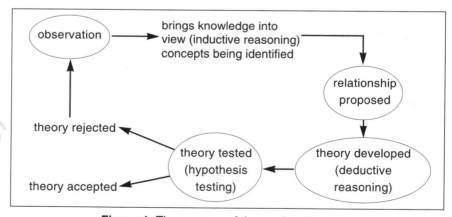

Figure 1: The process of theory development.

This model of theory development is reflected in the approach we adopt in research. An approach to research that draws on inductive reasoning is known as 'interpretative' or 'qualitative research'. This is contrasted with the approach to research which draws on deductive reasoning known as 'quantitative' or 'positivist' research. Each approach involves different ways of thinking about the world and exploring the world around us. (See *Figure 2*.)

	Qualitative research	Quantitative research
Also known as	interpretative	positivist
Knowledge at outset	little known	starts from a knowledge base
Type of reasoning	inductive reasoning	deductive reasoning
Link with concepts	identifies concepts	uses identified concepts and proposes relationship (theory)
Action	describes only	tests relationships between concepts (proposed theory) to look for facts
Outcome	brings knowledge to view may suggest relationships between concepts	accepts or rejects proposed theory

Figure 2: The broad distinction between qualitative and quantitative approaches to research.

Inductive reasoning can be seen as the first step in generating knowledge or identifying facts and it is the approach generally adopted by qualitative researchers.

Claire has worked for many years on a multi-disciplinary care team in the UK. One day she decides that she would like to find out more about the rest of the world and applies to work for an international care agency. She needs to find out as much as she can before going about the country she will be working in, partly for her own information, but also because she feels that the trip will offer her the opportunity to undertake some research about the culture in that country. When she is told about her placement Claire finds she has been allocated to work in a remote part of India.

ACTIVITY 8　　　　　　　ALLOW 5 MINUTES

List five things you think Claire might need to find out about India before she goes on her trip abroad and how she might find them out.

1

2

3

4

5

Commentary

In general we can assume that Claire might try to find out about:

- the climate (as this will affect the clothes she will take)

- appropriate dress style (should she always keep arms and legs covered, for example, so as not to offend cultural or religious sensitivities?)

- means of transport (will she need to consider providing her own transport?)

- economic situation and currency (what cash or type of travellers cheques will she need to take?)

- health risks (does she need to have any precautionary inoculations before leaving?)

- language and dialects spoken (does she need to find a phrase book or attempt to learn the basics of the language?).

By finding out these things Claire will be drawing on the *known facts* about the situation she is going to be working in. These facts would have been accrued over the years by a process of data collection and observations made by people who have visited that part of the world. This information is available in books, magazine articles, newspapers, films and documentaries.

With this information Claire can make some deductions about the culture, for example, deducing that because the climate has a high average temperature the weather will be hot. In this situation Claire has taken known facts about one situation and applied them to another situation. She knows that a country with a climatic temperature range of 25–30 degrees centigrade will be hot. This very simple example is being used to make clear a process which can be very complex when applying deductive reasoning to health and social care.

Now, what we need to do is to consider how Claire's research so far differs from other ways of finding out about the new culture. The known facts that are available have given Claire a good starting point, but have not provided all the information she requires. She might also want to understand the ways in which families relate to each other in India, how people feel about and live their religion, what they feel about work, and so on. She will probably have to find this out using inductive reasoning when she reaches the community she will be working in.

ACTIVITY 9   ALLOW 5 MINUTES

List three possible ways in which Claire might find out about the community and the people she will be working with when she arrives.

1

2

3

Commentary

1   When Claire goes to live in this new culture she will have the opportunity to absorb much of the activity that is going on around her by *observing* the local people at work, rest and play.

2   A second way would be to *talk* to as many people as possible – to ask them about their lifestyles, their beliefs, the factors that influence their life, and so on. She may, however, be limited by the number of people who can speak to her in English.

3   A third possible way is by reading the local newspapers and any other form of written material that is available, such as local official documents or historical documents.

4   Another possible source of data that spans both spoken and written words are the local stories passed down by story-tellers from generation to generation.

5   Finally, she could ask other members of the care agency team about their experiences and insights into this culture.

As a result of talking to people and observing the culture Claire will be able to build up a picture of the culture in which she is living and working. To gain acceptance into the culture Claire would also have to learn to speak the local language and be prepared to fit in with local customs and so on. In so doing she would be more able to draw on 'informal' sources of information – experiences drawn from every-day life rather than formalised, documented evidence about the situation. After a period of time, if little was known about this particular community, Claire could well become an authoritative source of information. In her case this source of information would have been derived from experience of the situation, observing what was happening and drawing knowledge into view – in other words from a process of inductive reasoning in which conclusions have been drawn based on that experience.

In summary, Claire would have three ways open to her of finding out about a country or situation: observing, talking and reading documents relating to the situation. We will now transfer the key points from this example to your own experience.

ACTIVITY 10   ALLOW 15 MINUTES

Consider any new situation you have found yourself in – for example, beginning school or college or starting a new job. How did you find out the facts about that situation and how did you find out how that culture worked?

1   List all the sources of *factual* information that were available to you.

2   List all the sources of *informal* information that were available to you

Commentary

1   You would probably have been given a range of factual information telling you about the environment you would be studying or working in. This could include maps of the environment and information sheets of organisational detail about colleagues and organisational structures. All of this would have given you a 'picture' of the organisation you were entering.

2   However, as you began to observe for yourself how the organisation worked, you probably began to get a deeper personal understanding of the processes that were outlined in the information sheets. Your own understanding would develop by actual observation of what was happening around you in that situation and by talking with your peer group or colleagues about their experiences in that organisation. The information sheets, for example, might state that all employees are seen as equals, but your own experiences might contradict this.

Researchers need to be alert to the potential limitations of their 'factual information' when trying to understand a situation more fully. Whilst factual information does provide an essential source of knowledge in the world we live in it may also serve to impede us from developing wider insights into the world around us unless we are also receptive to other sources of information. It is these other, non-factual sources of information which are so important in qualitative research.

Summary

1   In this session we have taken a broad overview of a number of issues, including consideration of how we develop knowledge, inductive and deductive reasoning and theory development.

2   Now we have explored these background issues about how we find out about the world, we can move on to consider how we might use this knowledge in developing our understanding of qualitative research.

Before you move on to Session Two, check that you have achieved the objectives given at the beginning of this session and, if not, review the appropriate sections.

Approaches to qualitative design

Introduction

In this session we will introduce a range of different approaches to qualitative research design and consider how these may be used. We will begin by exploring how qualitative and quantitative research design differs. We will then consider the basic ideas of using qualitative design for the purpose of exploration and description, before reviewing the use of qualitative research to interpret the world around us. We will explore qualitative research design from the perspective of:

- descriptive/exploratory research
- ethnography
- phenomenology
- grounded theory.

Session objectives

When you have completed this session you should be able to:

- describe the basic principles of qualitative design
- discuss a range of different approaches to qualitative research design
- match research questions to an appropriate research design

- explain what is meant by the term 'triangulation'

- discuss the concepts of validity and reliability in the context of qualitative research

- outline the potential ethical dilemmas researchers may face when completing qualitative research studies.

1: Principles of qualitative research

In the broadest terms, qualitative research is an approach that involves some kind of *interaction* between the researcher and the people or situation being researched and some form of *interpretation* of the situation. To do this, the researcher uses a process of *inductive reasoning*. Overall, it is an approach that helps us to draw some *meaning* out of a given situation.

Different authors emphasise different aspects of qualitative research in their definitions. For example, Brockup and Hastings-Tholsma (1995) state that 'qualitative research seeks to explore, describe or expand our knowledge of the world around us', while other authors put the emphasis on the study of individuals. 'Rather than testing preconceived ideas the researcher would seek to understand the issues from the point of view of the population being studied. Concepts and theories are generated from the respondents and emerge as the study progresses rather than the other way around.' (Clifford and Gough, 1990)

Silverman (1994) and Miles and Hubermans (1994) acknowledge the difficulties of adequately defining qualitative research. They define qualitative research as an umbrella term for a number of approaches with common features. These are that:

- the research seeks to establish a holistic perspective of the situation

- the research is conducted in 'real life', day-to-day situations

- the researcher attempts to identify the perceptions of the person being researched

- there is no single standardised way of collecting data

- the researcher uses small selective samples

- most analysis is done using words

- many interpretations of data are possible depending on the theoretical stance of the research

- the researcher may interact with the person being observed

- the researcher uses inductive reasoning

- the research is of low reliability but high validity

- no claims are made to generalise the findings.

To help you understand these features we will now contrast qualitative and quantitative research design.

2: Distinguishing qualitative from quantitative research design

The term **research design** refers to the overall plan for deciding how information is to be collected and analysed. It is this overall plan that determines the approach the researcher will adopt in the study.

Quantitative research approaches rely on objectivity – the researcher collects data in a way that is said to be 'distant from practice'. When research is referred to as having a 'quantitative orientation' it implies that some form of measurement or quantification is made in numerical terms. Broadly speaking, quantitative research approaches are *deductive*. Researchers start with something they know about and want to explore further. In applying numerical measures to data and using statistical techniques to analyse the results, researchers attempt to **generalise** their results to a wider population. To do this, they study a **random sample,** which means that every member of the population being studied has an equal chance of being studied. Such sampling techniques enable researchers to draw conclusions from the statistical tests performed and to make inferences about the findings for the rest of the population.

The purpose of qualitative research is to bring knowledge into view, so the approach reflects an *inductive* approach to research. In qualitative approaches the researcher commonly searches for meaning and insights in a given situation. The emphasis is on getting a holistic perspective of a situation and the research is conducted in 'real life' day-to-day situations. The data collected are in words, the medium by which most of us normally explain situations to ourselves.

Research design: *the overall plan for data collection and analysis in a research study.*

Generalisability: *the extent to which findings from a study sample can be generalised to the population from which the sample was taken.*

Random sample: *an approach to selecting a sample which ensures that each member of the population being studied has an equal chance of being selected.*

ACTIVITY 11 ALLOW 45 MINUTES

1 Read *Resource 1* in the *Resources Section*, an article by Carr (1994). Specifically written for nurses, the principles of qualitative and quantitative design are clearly covered.

2 When you have read the article, look at *Table 2* where you will see a list of the research design features discussed by Carr. Write down in the table a short summary of what Carr says about each approach, putting features of qualitative design in column A and features of quantitative design in column B.

	Column A Qualitative research	Column B Quantitative research
Type of reasoning used		
Historical influences		
Sampling		
Relationship of researcher with research		
Methods adopted		
Type of data		
Reliability		
Validity		
Ethical issues		

Table 2: Features of quantitative and qualitative research design.

Commentary

Your list of summarised points should be similar to that given in *Table 3*.

	Column A Qualitative research	Column B Quantitative research
Type of reasoning used	Inductive	Deductive
Historical influences	Seen as a subsidiary to quantitative research; primarily for discovery of knowledge to be tested	Traditionally accepted method; produces legitimate scientific answers
Sampling	In-depth nature of studies requires small selective samples	Requires random sample to undertake statistical tests and generalise findings
Relationship of researcher with research	Close, interactive relationship between researcher and subject	Researcher detached and distant from subject
Methods adopted	Ethnographic research grounded theory	Experimental/quasi-experimental; correlational; descriptive
Type of data	'Soft' – words rather than numbers	'Hard' data presented in numerical form and subject to statistical testing

	Column A Qualitative research	Column B Quantitative research
Reliability	Lack of standardisation makes reliability difficult to assess	More reliable as eliminates extraneous variables
Validity	Has validity as conducted in natural setting	More difficult to determine validity if not in natural setting
Ethical issues to be considered	Safety and protection of human rights. Hard to determine informed consent when working in unknown area	Safety and protection of human rights. Risk in formulating hypothesis

Table 3: Comparison of quantitative and qualitative research.

3: Sampling methods in qualitative research

As we know, qualitative research is conducted in 'real life', day-to-day situations. The research is carried out using small, select sample groups. This is variously described as:

- purposive sampling
- theoretical sampling
- opportunistic sampling
- snowball sampling.

In **purposive sampling** the sample is selected purposively on the basis of a particular variable that is being studied. The same principle is used in **theoretical sampling**, a term used by some qualitative researchers to indicate that sample selection is driven by the theoretical basis of the study. In **opportunistic sampling** the researcher selects a sample simply as the opportunity presents itself, using the principles of purposive and/or theoretical sampling to identify the sample. **Snowball sampling** arises from this. When a researcher identifies one respondent he or she might ask if the respondent knows any other people who might fit the sampling requirement and a snowballing effect is created.

Sample size in qualitative research

The sample size used in qualitative research is generally much smaller than in quantitative research. In qualitative research the researcher is looking for *meaning* in the data, rather than trying to get an appropriate sample to enable statistical testing to determine whether the findings could be generalised to the wider situation. It is not uncommon for research reports of qualitative studies to report on very small numbers of respondents. When you read qualitative research reports you will see references to **saturation** of data. This means that the researcher may start without any predetermined sample size and will continue to collect data until new ideas cease to emerge.

Purposive/theoretical sampling: *a sampling technique used in qualitative research in which the researcher chooses the sample on the basis of known characteristics or experiences.*

Opportunistic sampling: *the researcher selects a sample simply as the opportunity presents itself, using the principles of purposive/theoretical sampling to identify the sample.*

Snowball sampling: *arises from opportunistic sampling. When a researcher identifies one respondent he or she asks whether the respondent knows any other people who might meet the sampling requirement.*

Saturation: *the point at which the researcher gathering and analysing qualitative data feels that no new categories are emerging.*

23

In qualitative research there is no single, standardised way of collecting data – the method will be determined by what the researcher wants to find out. Generally the researcher will interact with the person or people being studied, either by interviewing or by observing what they are doing. Whichever method is used, the data are collected in words rather than in figures.

Many interpretations of data are possible, depending on the theoretical stance of the researcher. It is this last point that we are concerned about in the rest of this session and we now go on to explore it further.

4: Different approaches to qualitative research

Researchers using a qualitative approach might approach their work in a number of different ways. We will begin by considering the situation where a researcher might use the broad principles of qualitative research to explore or *describe* a situation. We will then look at the various ways a researcher might approach the interpretation of data collected in a qualitative research design.

Descriptive design

Data collected using qualitative approaches can be used in two ways:

- to *describe* or *explore* the situation by summarising findings

- to *interpret* situations.

For example, when gathering descriptive data we might ask people to tell us in their own words what they feel about living in the UK today. When we analyse those data we might simply report what people stated in a summary format. This differs from interpreting the data where we would endeavour to explain what we are seeing.

Descriptive or exploratory design is a very commonly used approach to research, in which the researcher simply wants to explore or identify what is going on in a given situation – as shown in the following scenario.

In a small town in the Midlands, a group of health and social workers have identified many anomalies in the allocation of resources for health and social care. For example, it appeared that more resources were being allocated to one area than to others that were equally in need, simply because that had historically always been the case. It also appeared that clients were being shunted from one service to another without any clear idea of who was responsible for their care. Clients were constantly referred between both social and health care groups, monitored by separate records and subject to duplication of effort. The group felt that the way funding for care provision was allocated, together with poor communication channels, meant that they were duplicating services and using resources in a way that was service-driven rather than driven by the needs of the client.

Once these problems had been identified, the group decided to establish a new programme of care provision in which the needs of the clients directed the use of resources. To do this they developed a collaborative

---

assessment system that could be completed either by the social worker or by the nursing or paramedical staff. The managers ensured that all the staff were appropriately trained in the new system, which was implemented at the beginning of the year.

After the new system had been in operation for almost a year the managers monitored its progress using a regular auditing mechanism. The audit data indicated that staff were able to keep a closer track on clients in their care and were able to monitor their progress through the support systems quickly and efficiently. However, the managers came to realise that although the new system was having a positive impact in terms of the quantifiable data collected, no one had asked the clients what they actually thought about it.

Two members of the team were allocated to undertake a research study in which they were to find out clients' views of the new service. As it was a new service the team members felt that a qualitative approach would be more appropriate than a quantitative one. They would be able to use open-ended interview questions to focus their enquiry, gathering data using face-to-face interviews in which they would write the responses down as the interview progressed.

The team members devised an interview schedule (an open-ended questionnaire) which used five short open-ended questions to focus their enquiry.

Interview schedule:

1 Please can you tell me about care you have been receiving?

2 Is this care meeting your expectations – if 'yes' why? if 'no' why not?

3 Is it an improvement on previous care – if 'yes' why? if 'no' why not?

4 Are the people from the health and social service agencies responding to your requests for care?

5 Do you have any suggestions about ways in which we could improve our care?

ACTIVITY 12   ALLOW 5 MINUTES

Think of a situation relevant to your own work environment in which it might be appropriate for you to undertake a descriptive/exploratory qualitative research study similar to that described above.

Commentary

If you are working in health and social care there might be a number of dimensions of care-giving that would lend themselves to this approach. They might be to do with exploring aspects of satisfaction with a particular service offered. For example, nurse-led outpatient clinics are being introduced in the NHS to replace clinics traditionally held by medical staff and the question here would be whether patients are satisfied with the care in such clinics. Another example would be an evaluation of new treatment, such as a new rehabilitation programme.

Interpretative design

The three most common approaches to interpretative design are:

- ethnography

- phenomenology

- grounded theory.

All three are now used in health and social care research. The important distinction between these approaches lies in the way researchers view the world. The origin of each approach comes from three different theoretical perspectives or schools of thinking (see *Table 4*). We will look at each in turn.

Type of research design	Theoretical influences
Ethnography	Anthropology
Phenomenology	Philosophy
Grounded theory	Sociology

Table 4: Types of research design and theoretical influences.

These three approaches to research use inductive reasoning in that they aim to bring knowledge into view. However, the particular perspective from which they seek to do this will vary according to orientation.

Ethnography

*Ethnography:
an approach to research influenced by the anthropological tradition, in which the researcher seeks to understand human behaviour from the perspective of the individual in a given culture.*

Ethnography focuses on the description of culture and can be defined as a 'generalised approach to developing concepts to understand human behaviour' (Field and Morse, 1996). It can be useful in health and social care in trying to understand the influences in and practices of a particular culture. Ethnography reflects the theoretical perspective of anthropology, the study of people in natural conditions, either by directly observing individuals or groups, or by tracing the origins of that group.

What the anthropologist is trying to do is to understand the world of the culture being observed. For the researcher who plans to do an ethnographic study, the research will involve collecting data which describe the culture under study. A researcher following this tradition may use many methods to collect information. These might include:

- interviews and observation

- use of records

- tracing historical facts such as life histories

- referring to other documented evidence such as news reports or diaries.

There are many strong arguments in favour of using this approach in health and social care. After all, if we have a clearer understanding of the culture of the client groups that we are working with it should help us to direct our care to meet their needs more appropriately. To illustrate this we will now consider a situation where a health worker wishes to use an ethnographic approach to research.

ACTIVITY 13   ALLOW 20 MINUTES

Read the scenario below and write down in the space below it the ways in which Matthew could collect data for his study.

> **Matthew** is a nurse working with a general practitioner in a busy inner-city surgery. Whilst he deals with his day-to-day work very efficiently he feels that his own education and background have not really prepared him to fully understand what it is like to be a patient using the community health care provision in this inner-city area. He feels that if he could understand better he would be able to improve the quality of the care he gives. He is particularly concerned about those people from various ethnic minority groups who come to the surgery. The mix of clients includes a large group of elderly people of Polish origin, as well as members of Vietnamese and Asian communities.
>
> Matthew is given an opportunity to undertake a research study as part of his own professional development. He decides to use this to try and understand the patients' cultures. He plans an ethnographic study in which he will explore what it is like to be a patient. He wants to do this from an ethnographic perspective and when planning his study he entitles it 'the waiting room culture'. He feels that the mix of people from different backgrounds attending the surgery provides an unusual cultural mix that might not be readily available in another situation.

Commentary

Data for an ethnographic study such as this could be collected by:

- observation

- interviews

- use of records that might indicate patterns of attendance or specific health problems.

Matthew's sample will comprise any people participating in that culture who attend the surgery. All may be involved in some way in the data collected by observation, but Matthew might be more selective when choosing a smaller sample for interviews.

Of course, as with all research methods Matthew could not just go straight ahead and carry out his research. He would first need to get permission to undertake it, both from the responsible managers and from a local ethical committee. This is because at all times when completing research we must ensure that the privacy and dignity of the people we are working with are not undermined.

Ethical issues in qualitative research

Ethical issues are mainly concerned with a balance between protecting the rights of people for privacy, safety, confidentiality and protection from deceit, whilst at the same time pursuing scientific endeavour. As we work through the rest of this text we will refer to the need for researchers to take care that they do not infringe any human rights when collecting or analysing data in a research study. As you will see, in qualitative research we are often working in unknown territory and so it is not always so easy to be able to state exactly what we plan to do in our studies. For example, it is harder to describe to an external agency what will be done in a phenomenological study. This can cause specific problems to researchers undertaking qualitative research – problems that are not so apparent in quantitative research because it is much more structured and focused.

In another title in this series (Clifford et al., 1997) we considered in depth some of the ethical issues that face researchers. The important point to remember here is that in health care all research projects, no matter how small, must be approved by a local ethics committee. It is the researcher's task to demonstrate that any potential ethical issues involved in the research are justified by the importance of the research in the pursuit of knowledge and potential improvement in client care.

Let us assume that, having got permission to proceed, Matthew collects the data using a combination of observation, interviews and reference to patient records as appropriate.

ACTIVITY 14   ALLOW 10 MINUTES

Look back at *Table 2* showing the list of attributes of qualitative design. Describe those aspects of qualitative design listed below which you think Matthew's study might be using.

- Type of reasoning

- Sampling procedure

- Relationship between researcher and subjects

- Methods adopted

- Type of data

- Ethical issues

Commentary

Your summary should look something like that shown in *Table 5*.

Features of qualitative design	Factors in this study
Inductive/deductive reasoning	Inductive
Sampling	Constrained by patients available in the waiting room
Relationship of researcher with subjects	Direct contact in the waiting room
Methods adopted	Observation; interviews; records
Type of data	Words – generated through interview, observation notes and records
Ethical issues	Potential risk of invading privacy Would need to get permission

Table 5: Factors related to qualitative research design in Matthew's study.

The study is inductive as Matthew is wanting to uncover new facts about the culture. The sampling is clearly limited to patients in the locality and the researcher will have direct contact with them in the waiting room. If observation and interview methods are adopted, Matthew will relate directly with his subjects.

In summary, we have seen that ethnography is an approach to research that focuses on the study of culture with the aim of understanding how that culture works. This involves the researcher collecting data by observation and interview, in addition to using any other available records that might support the research. Insights about specific cultures provided through ethnography can help health and social workers to manage the situations they are in. Morse (1992) has brought together a series of classic papers relating to the ethnographic approach to illustrate this, including ethnographic study of care provision in nursing homes, the role of surgeons, and a study of the mental hospital cult.

Phenomenology

Phenomenology has its roots in philosophy, an influence that emphasises the subjectivity of human experiences and behaviour. The researcher using a phenomenological approach is interested in finding out the meaning of a given situation *to the participant.* Field and Morse (1996) suggest that phenomenology 'guides one back from theoretical abstraction to the reality of lived experience' leaving the phenomenologist free to ask the question 'What is it like to have a certain experience?'

Phenomenological research, then, is directed towards active involvement in one person's reality – for example, what it means to be a person waiting for a cardiac transplant (which may be his or her only remaining source of hope for life) or what it is like to be a nurse or a social worker in the 1990s. Field and Morse (1996) suggest that phenomenologists never reach a conclusion but that, in asking the question 'what is it like for you?', the phenomenologist will be challenging the reader to say 'yes, it is like this', or 'no, I do not believe it is like this'.

To help develop the interpretation of the situation being studied, the phenomenological researcher may draw on other sources of data, such as novels, films or researching other people's research. As we saw in Session One, these are all influences that help to shape our knowledge. For example, a phenomenological researcher asking what it is like to be a nurse would interview nurses about their experiences but might also look at the many films, books and other media portrayals of nurses in order to help them understand 'what it is like to be a nurse'.

As the focus in phenomenological research is on *individual* meanings, the sample selection method used is different to that used in studying a culture in an ethnographic study. The researcher has to identify a sample of people who will be able to participate because they have personal experience of the phenomenon under study.

In the case study below, Aiden, the social worker, is going to undertake a study of young offenders. Since he is asking the question 'What does it mean be a young offender?' and wants to understand this from the young offender's point of view, there would be little value in him searching out a sample group of people who are not young offenders. He will therefore only seek out youngsters classed as young offenders. This is an example of purposive sampling. People who will participate in the study will be identified on the basis of their experience of the subject being studied.

Aiden is a social worker who works with young offenders. He is concerned that he has little insight into what makes these youngsters into offenders and feels that if he could understand this more he would be able to help his clients better and possibly reduce the level of offending in his client group. His research question is 'What is it like to be a young offender?'

Aiden sets about establishing his study by identifying a small group of teenagers who have been labelled as 'young offenders', on the basis of a track record of problems with the law. He asks them whether they would be willing to participate in this study and then proceeds to collect his data through a series of in-depth interviews with this group.

Once he has gathered his interview data he proceeds to analyse them to try and understand what these youngsters feel about being classed as 'young offenders'. To help in his interpretation he also draws on

---

literature, newspaper articles, films and documentary programes which address this issue from different perspectives. These sources contribute to his understanding and interpretation of the data he has gathered from young offenders who responded to his question 'What is it like to be a young offender?'

ACTIVITY 15	ALLOW 5 MINUTES

Think of a situation in your own working experience in which it could be useful to use a phenomenological perspective.

Commentary

Obviously your response to this will depend on your own working situation and you may have come up with quite a long list or only a very short one. You might, for example, want to know what it means to belong to a particular minority group in society. Depending on your perspective and caring role, this could include considering what it is like to be disabled, chronically ill, unemployed or elderly and infirm. Alternatively, you could look at this from a professional perspective and consider what it means be a care assistant, a nurse or a social worker.

Phenomenology focuses on the 'lived experience' of the individual. The phenomenological researcher endeavours to stand aside from a situation and ensure that the focus of the collection and analysis of data is on the individual under study.

Grounded theory

The purpose of **grounded theory** is to unearth the *social processes* involved in the subject being studied. The major theoretical influence on this approach is sociology. Field and Morse (1996) point out that this approach can be seen as broadly similar to other qualitative approaches in terms of data collection, but that it is a more 'process orientated' approach. It seeks to unravel the elements of an experience and to challenge the elements or theoretical concepts as they emerge in the data by looking for alternative cases. (This is known as the 'constant comparison method'.) Theory is generated as the research progresses to explain how those concepts fit together, causing the researcher to follow leads and to develop ideas during the research to ensure that the theory is grounded in the data (Strauss and Corbin, 1990).

Grounded theory: *an approach to research in which the aim is to collect and analyse qualitative data in order to develop theory which is 'grounded' in the data.*

Grounded theory is rather different to the other approaches discussed so far, because it uses both inductive and deductive reasoning. The researcher formulates tentative theories about what is observed (using inductive reasoning) and then follows up these ideas by further enquiry (deductive reasoning). Although this approach may seem to be contrary to our description of the distinction between qualitative and quantitative research, in using inductive *and* deductive reasoning the researcher using grounded theory is aiming both to unearth new knowledge and to propose new theories. Thus, grounded theory falls into the category of generation of knowledge through *theory development* rather than theory testing. It is therefore categorised as a qualitative approach to research in a number of texts.

The sampling procedure in grounded theory is described as 'theoretical sampling' (Strauss and Corbin, 1990). The researcher may change direction as the research progresses to follow up ideas as theory emerges and evolves.

The approach to data analysis in grounded theory is more structured than in other methods (Field and Morse, 1996). Data is analysed concurrently as it is collected. Once the basic social processes have been clarified the researcher can claim the ideas that have been generated from the research, but then will turn to other sources of data to support or reject the emerging ideas. Thus, this approach relies more heavily on other sources of research than ethnographic or phenomenological perspectives (Field and Morse, 1996).

This wide perspective allows the researcher to change direction and to pursue ideas as they arise in the data. Any text guiding researchers through this process will discuss the **constant comparison method** of analysis – in which the researcher looks for patterns in the data. Any emerging theories that arise out of the research are said to be *grounded* in the data.

This can all sound very complicated and, indeed, the grounded theory approach is not to be recommended to the newcomer to research. Nevertheless, to illustrate its use let us consider a study in which a researcher wishes to examine the social unit of the family using a grounded theory approach.

The study involves an initial round of interviews focusing on people who belong to an identified family unit, a husband, wife and two children. As a result of this initial study the researcher concludes that a key process involved in the family situation is marriage, which is indicative of the groups studied thus far. However, the researcher wishes to look for the 'alternative case' to compare whether marriage is actually a key process in creating a family unit. The factors promoting this new line of thought come from literature and the media, which indicate that a large number of families in the West have not undergone conventional marriage ceremonies.

A second round of interviews is undertaken, with families which have not gone through a wedding ceremony. As a result of this second round of interviews, the researcher is beginning to identify other features or 'processes' that contribute towards a description of the family unit. For example, regardless of whether the couples had completed a wedding ceremony all exhibited a commitment to each other. The concept of commitment therefore emerges as a point of focus for the next line of enquiry. This second step is identified as a 'core' process but, as with the first, there is a need to challenge it and look for the alternative case to provide a point of comparison; namely to ask whether there are any families that do *not* exhibit this commitment. The study progresses from here as the researcher tries to identify other subsidiary processes involved in family life with which to provide an explanatory network of relationships.

The following scenario gives a second example of a grounded theory approach.

> **Iona** is a health visitor working with single-parent families in the community. She is concerned that the young children of these parents seems to be having difficulty relating to people outside their small family unit (inductive reasoning). She decides to study this problem using a grounded theory approach. She chooses a sample of ten single-parent families in which the children are between five and ten years old. She proceeds with her investigation by observing the interaction between child and parent in the clinic and at school.
>
> As the study progresses, Iona analyses the data for common patterns and emerging themes (inductive reasoning). On the basis of these observations she draws on her knowledge of parenting (deductive reasoning) and formulates some tentative theories about how the parents and children cope with their relationships outside the small family unit. She proceeds to develop an interview schedule to explore these tentative theories and interviews the single parents about this.
>
> As the data analysis progresses it starts to indicate clear trends in the pattern of relationships with parents and children in a single-parent situation. This leads Iona to formulate a tentative theory about levels of dependency between parent and child in single parent units (deductive reasoning drawing on known theories of dependency). However, to check if this theory can be supported Iona needs to return to research literature to explore the previous work that has been undertaken on child-parent relationships. This allows her to formulate a theory about how the relationship between parent and child in a single-parent family influences the way the child relates to others outside the family.

Since Iona was only using a small sample in her study, she can state that her findings are grounded in the data she has collected through the study, but she cannot claim that the findings from the study can be generalised to the whole population. To verify this new theory Iona will need to study other single-parent families to determine whether the patterns of relationships she has proposed in her theory can be supported.

ACTIVITY 16   ALLOW 10 MINUTES

Think of an area in your own work in which a grounded theory approach would be an appropriate means of study.

Commentary

The emphasis in a grounded theory approach is on uncovering the sociological processes that impact on different facets of life. Examples might include:

- the working relationships between health and social care teams
- understanding why people expose themselves to health risks such as the risks from smoking, alcohol, and drugs
- understanding why people react as they do in certain social situations.

In grounded theory data are analysed as they emerge using inductive reasoning. This allows the researcher to explore new ideas as they emerge in the study. Then, if appropriate, the researcher can follow up other ideas using the emerging theory and established knowledge from other sources such as the literature (deductive reasoning).

Matching the research question to the design

As we have seen, qualitative research can be divided into two categories—descriptive or exploratory research and interpretative research approaches, using ethnography, phenomenology and grounded theory. If you have a relatively clear grasp of the orientation of each of these approaches to research then it is quite easy to match the question to the design.

For example, if we were undertaking a study in which we were looking for the meaning of a particular experience to an individual we would not do an observation study as this would tell us very little about how an individual *feels*. Similarly, if we wanted to look at a culture we would need to observe the *groups* in that culture and not just the individuals. As the researcher establishes the focus of the research or asks the research question the appropriate design to answer that question becomes more apparent.

ACTIVITY 17   ALLOW 10 MINUTES

Look at the list of research examples below. Below each example note which research approach would be appropriate and state your reasons.

1 What are clients' views about the Community Care Act?

2 What does it mean to be a social worker in Britain in the 1990s?

3 A study of the inner-city culture of street children.

4   What are the social factors influencing health and social care organisation in the UK?

Commentary

1   The question could be a descriptive qualitative study because it focuses simply on views which could be interpreted at a descriptive level of study.

2   This question could be a phenomenological study because it uses the word 'mean', which has implications of meaning to the individual.

3   A study of children in the inner-city could be an ethnographic study because the focus of the question is on the inner-city culture.

4   This question could be a grounded theory study because the question asks about social factors.

5: Reliability and validity in qualitative research

Traditionally, researchers from different disciplines have placed great emphasis on the concepts of **reliability** and **validity** in research. Reliability refers to a concept in research in which any measurement tool that we use consistently measures the same features whilst validity is the extent to which a research tool measures what it is supposed to measure.

In designing research studies these aspects must be considered carefully. As Carr indicated in the paper you read in *Resource 1*, there are differences here between quantitative and qualitative research. Researchers using quantitative research try to ensure that the instruments they use to collect data are reliable by removing any **extraneous variables** – any variables other than the independent variable which may influence the effect to be measured.

When designing research tools such as questionnaires, researchers using quantitative approaches spend long periods of time developing and refining their questionnaires to ensure that responses will be reliable. They can do this in several ways. One of these is a simple **test–re-test** approach.

This allows the researcher to administer a questionnaire to a group of respondents on one occasion and then, perhaps several weeks later, administer the same questionnaire to the same group of respondents. The researcher then looks for consistency in the two sets of responses. If most of the respondents do not answer in the same way as they did on the first occasion, the researcher might assume either that they have changed their views or that the way in which the questions are phrased does not generate a consistent interpretation. It is more likely that the latter reason would account for inconsistency, because it is unlikely that a range of people would all change their views on a given topic over a short period of time.

In qualitative research we are asking people to describe things in their own words. The nature of the response we get is therefore likely to be different.

Reliability:
the ability of a measurement procedure to produce the same results when used in different places by different researchers. An example of this could be a ruler – this reliably measures length regardless of when, where or who is using it.

Validity:
the extent to which a research tool measures what it is supposed to measure.

Extraneous variable:
any variable other than the independent variable which may influence the effect to be measured.

Therefore, we could not claim that our questions were going to result in the same or consistent responses from all respondents. Because the instruments used for collecting data in qualitative research do not yield consistent responses, reliability in qualitative research is said to be low compared with highly structured, quantitative questionnaires.

In qualitative research, however, it is easier to measure what is supposed to be measured and therefore validity is said to be high in qualitative research. Although quantitative research tools may gather consistent responses, highly structured approaches make it harder to be sure that we are measuring what we are supposed to measure – to guarantee validity. Quantitative researchers will spend a long period of time developing tools to ensure they address the issue of validity. For the qualitative researcher, however, this can be much more straightforward. For example, if we were to ask a group of people to tell us what they felt about the National Health Service today we might anticipate the sorts of things they would say. If trying to get the same information by structured questionnaire we would need to take care not to anticipate the responses in the way in which we phrased the questions.

There are also some additional ways in which we can check the validity of our data in qualitative research. We can refer back to the person interviewed and ask him or her to check the way we have interpreted his or her response by asking 'does this interpretation ring true for you?'. If the interpretation is considered inaccurate then we can review our procedures for selection of ideas and concepts and reconsider the data.

6: Triangulation

Triangulation:
the use of more than one method of collecting or interpreting data. For example, using observation and interviews, or structured questionnaires and interviews.

Triangulation is the use of both quantitative and qualitative methods of collecting or analysing data in order to get a more accurate picture of what is going on. The value of triangulation can be demonstrated by referring back to Matthew's study in the doctor's surgery. Here we said that Matthew may collect data by using observation, interviews and by looking at records. Collecting data using a mixed methodological approach will give him a much richer picture of the situation he is studying. He is able to validate his data by observing what was happening in the surgery, by asking people what they felt and by using data to focus on the same issue. Had he used only one of these techniques of data collection his research would have been lacking in the depth and richness that the multiple perspectives offer.

In our reference to reliability above, we noted that a researcher might use a questionnaire to ask people to respond to questions attempting to establish their views of the National Health Service. If this was followed up by a qualitative-orientated interview, the researcher would then be getting a much deeper picture of the respondents' views. The researcher could gather the views of a larger respondent group in quantitative terms as well as the more in-depth analysis generated by a smaller number of in-depth interviews.

Summary

1   In this session we have looked at the basic principles of qualitative design. We have considered a number of related issues.

2   We have looked at the principles of qualitative research that take account of different forms of interaction between researchers and their subjects and how this interaction is interpreted.

3   We have explored the features that distinguish qualitative and quantitative design. The notion of design has been considered with particular reference to the collection and analysis of information.

4   Sampling methods and their different approaches to the identification of a research population have been examined.

5   The complexities associated with reliability and validity in the collection and measurement of data have been reviewed and ethical issues and the rights of the people who form the research population discussed.

Before you move on to Session Three you should check that you have achieved the objectives given at the beginning of this session and, if not, review the appropriate sections.

Collecting data in qualitative design

Introduction

In this session we will be exploring the use of interview and observation techniques in data collection. We will look at the general approaches adopted in both forms of data collection and the strengths and weaknesses of each. We will then discuss the use of other records, such as diaries and historical records, as sources of data in qualitative research design.

Session objectives

When you have completed this session you should be able to:

- identify when it is appropriate to use interview techniques to collect data

- explain the stages involved in collecting data via interviews

- discuss the strengths and weaknesses of the interview approach

- establish when it is appropriate to use observation techniques to collect data

- outline how data can be collected through observation

- describe the strengths and weaknesses of the observational approach.

1: Using interviews in qualitative research

Interview techniques are widely used as a means of gathering data in qualitative research. For many people working in health and social care, conducting interviews does not create any anxiety, probably because our day-to-day work involves us in various forms of interviews with patients and clients. By the same token this means that health workers may fail to fully appreciate the implications of interviews carried out for research purposes. When using interviews in their daily work health workers usually interview one individual about one subject. However, in research we are usually trying to gather information on the same topic from more than one respondent, and this makes the process more complex.

There are several ways in which interviews can be conducted, as you probably know from your own experience. Before we go any further it would be useful for you to review your own experience of being interviewed, whether for a new job, as part of someone else's research project or in a market research survey.

ACTIVITY 18　　　　　　　　　ALLOW **10** MINUTES

1　List as many occasions as you can remember on which you have been interviewed.

2　Looking at your list, consider the ways in which these interviews differed in style. Were you expected to answer a simple 'yes' or 'no' to questions, or were you required to comment in some depth?

Commentary

1　Your list might contain any of the following:

- an interview when you started a new college course or a new job

- periodic interviews with teachers or managers reviewing your progress on a course or at work

- an interview when you were stopped in the street and asked your views on a particular product or political party

- an interview by a member of the press

- a group interview in which you participated.

2　Given the range of possible interview situations there are, you have probably experienced several kinds of interviews. For example, if you have ever been stopped by a market researcher in the street you may have noted that he or she worked through a highly structured interview questionnaire which required specific answers such as 'yes', 'no' or 'don't know' (for example, 'Do you use margarine X?').

Other interview questions you've experienced may have been less structured. For example, an interviewer may have had a set of questions they were working to, but rather than asking you to respond to a prescribed response (such as 'yes','no', 'don't know') they may have asked you to describe something in your own words by saying 'Tell me what you think of our products...'. This semi-structured interview style is often used by people undertaking interviews for jobs because they want to give all candidates the opportunity to comment on the same topics but not restrict questions to 'yes/no' answers which wouldn't help the interviewer discover much about the candidate.

You may also have experienced an interview in which the person interviewing you did not appear to be working to set questions at all but instead seemed to be holding a conversation with you. This is described as an open interview.

Types of interview

Several approaches may be taken to interviews, ranging from a highly structured through a semi-structured to a very low-structured (open) approach. Each approach is characterised by a different format for the questions asked and the sequence in which the questions are administered – as indicated in *Table 6*. The choice of approach used will depend on the research design. For example, if you were doing a quantitative survey you would use a highly structured interview and if you were doing a qualitative study you might use a semi-structured or a low-structured one.

Highly structured	Semi-structured	Low structured
● structured questions	● focused questions	● open questions
● fixed order/sequence of questioning	● sequence of questioning may vary	● conversational approach – no prescribed sequence
● data can be analysed numerically	● data transcribed into words	● data transcribed into words

Table 6: Summary of approaches to interviews.

ACTIVITY 19   ALLOW 10 MINUTES

Read the three case studies below and then:

a) Indicate the kind of interview approach you think has been adopted in each.

b) Draw on your knowledge from the previous session to indicate the type of qualitative research approach that has been adopted.

Type of interview	Type of research
Case study 1:	
Case study 2:	
Case study 3:	

Case study 1

Katherine is the manager of an opticians which has a shop selling spectacles and eye care solutions. She has been asked by her regional manager to find out the clients' views of the service offered. She is particularly interested in identifying what customers think about the speed and efficiency of the service. Katherine decides that she will construct a questionnaire asking people to respond to a checklist identifying different aspects of the services provided in the shop. She decides to use this questionnaire to interview a sample made up of every tenth person to enter the shop during the following week. She considers that in this way she will get a fairly representative sample of shop users.

Katherine uses the following questions:

Please indicate the extent to which you use our service.	a lot	a little
Do you feel the service meets your needs?	yes	no
Do you use other shops which provide the same services?	yes	no

Case study 2

Daniel is a social worker working in an elderly care team. His managers have asked him to undertake some research to answer two questions. The first is to explore the frequency and length of visits elderly clients receive from social workers in the team. The second is to find out what the elderly clients feel about the service that is being offered.

Daniel is faced with the challenge of deciding how to collect this data. He knows that some parts of this research could be answered by using a questionnaire, but he also recognises that some of his clients would have difficulty completing a questionnaire – either because their eyesight was poor or because they had other problems such as arthritis which would interfere with their ability to write. He also feels he would be better placed to ask clients what they feel about the service if he could meet with people face to face. He therefore develops an interview schedule that is divided into two parts. The first part asks the elderly people to indicate:

● how frequently they have been visited by a social worker in the last month

● how long the social worker stayed with them on each visit.

The second part of the questionnaire uses the following question to get the elderly people to say what they think about the social services:

'Tell me in your own words what you think of the social services.'

> ## Case study 3
>
> **Andrew** is a paramedic working in a big city. He is doing a degree course in which he is required to undertake a small research project. When considering what he would like to research he decided he would like to try answering the question 'What does it feel like to be a victim of a road traffic accident?' He therefore decided he would develop a qualitative research study to address this question. Andrew decided to interview people who had been the victim of a road accident in the previous year. As no other researchers had undertaken a similar study before he felt that he would like to approach this by simply asking the participants one question, 'How did you feel following the road accident?' and then allowing the interview to take a normal, conversational shape.

Commentary

a) Case study 1 is a highly structured interview in which Katherine is asking respondents to give responses to very specific questions.

Case study 2 is a mixture of highly structured and semi-structured. The first questions are very specific, but the last one is designed to get the interviewees to respond to a specific area in their own words and is therefore semi-structured.

Case study 3 is an open interview in which Andrew is trying to get 'meaning' from a conversational style interview.

b) Both Case study 1 and Case study 2 are descriptive exploratory studies. Case study 3, although not clearly stated, could be described as a phenomenological approach, as Andrew is trying to understand what it feels like to be a victim of a road traffic accident.

2: Constructing and carrying out interviews in research

In using interviews in research it is possible to identify three stages:

1   the planning stage

2   the 'doing' stage, conducting the interview

3   the analysis stage.

We will look at each of these in turn.

Planning interviews

At the planning stage you will be making the fundamental decisions about the way you are going to approach your research work. It is very easy when starting out in research to think that, because you have a good idea for an interview, it will therefore work well. However, as with all aspects of life, a little careful planning is usually necessary in order to avoid the pitfalls of interviews into which you might stumble.

There are a number of aspects you need to consider:

- who you are going to interview

- the structure of the interview

- the structure of the questions *within* the interview

- how to collect the information

- how to relate to the people being interviewed (the interviewees).

We have already discussed the first two of these points. When we discussed sampling in Session Two we noted that qualitative researchers can select a purposive sample, that is, people who have experience of the particular phenomenon under study. For example, a study asking people about experiences of health care would be pretty useless if undertaken with people who had no experience of health care systems.

The various approaches to interviews have also been described. As you will recall, a highly structured interview is one in which the researcher asks fixed questions which have a limited range of potential responses – in other words, closed questions. A semi-structured interview allows the researcher more scope by establishing a focus to the questions but leaving the style of responding entirely to the respondents. A low-structured approach is the most conversational style of interview. We will now look a little more closely at the kind of questions that can be asked in each approach.

Question structure

A researcher completing a highly structured interview survey of people's experiences of health care will ask respondents closed questions such as 'Were you satisfied with your treatment?' or 'Would you choose to return to this centre for follow-up care?' Such questions invite a fixed response of 'yes', 'no' or 'don't know'. This is why they are referred to as **closed questions.**

Closed question: *the kind of question in which a researcher expects a limited range of responses. Contrasts with an open question.*

Open question: *a way of phrasing a question to gather data from respondents in a research study. The question requires the respondent to make an individual response. For example, the researcher may ask 'Please tell me what you think about ...'. Contrasts with a closed question.*

A semi-structured interview question approach gives the researcher more flexibility in the range of potential responses. For example, a researcher might ask respondents 'Can you tell me what you think about the care you received?' or 'Can you tell me why you chose to come to this centre for your care?' Such questions may be one of a series asking people to give their views about health care. They have some structure, in that the focus of the question is clear to the respondents, but as they are not limited to a range of responses they will reply in their own words. Because these questions have a focus the researcher can anticipate a limited range of responses being given. For example, a patient responding to the question 'Can you tell me what you think about the care you received?' may, depending on his or her experience, state that he or she felt very satisfied or very dissatisfied with the care received. The benefit in using this approach over the closed question approach is that in this situation the respondent can elaborate on his or her response and perhaps offer reasons for the way he or she feels.

A low-structured interview question might simply state an opening remark, for example, 'I am interested in your experience of health care – can we talk about it?' The interviewer then uses a normal conversational style, perhaps using prompts to keep the focus of the questions on the topic.

Collecting the information

The two most common ways of collecting information from an interview are writing it down or using a tape recorder. Writing down the responses is the logical choice with highly structured questions and, to some extent, with semi-structured interviews. However, once the volume of data generated in an interview starts to increase it can be quite hard to keep up. Writing down information can in itself become a block to communication, because a researcher concentrating on writing cannot concentrate on communicating. The tape recorder or video might therefore seem to be a better option for interviewing than writing. However, whilst tape-recorders or videos may be preferred by the researcher, they can be seen as intrusive by the person being interviewed.

Relating to the interviewees

Another point to be considered in the planning stage is how the researcher will relate to the people to be interviewed. First, there is a need to consider how respondents will be contacted in the first instance. Will potential interviewees be approached and told about the project face to face, or will the researcher send a letter telling them about the project and asking for volunteers? There may be concerns, especially in health and social care situations, that people could feel coerced into participating and, in ethical terms, sending a letter would probably be considered less intrusive.

What to tell respondents about the study is another planning issue. In qualitative research this matter requires quite a lot of consideration. For example, a researcher undertaking a phenomenological study on people's feelings about drug taking may not want to go into a lot of detail in an information letter in case they pass on their own ideas to potential respondents. As every study will have its own unique orientation the best advice for beginner researchers at this stage is to ask an advisor or supervisor for help.

Other general communication issues, such as how you will introduce yourself to the people being interviewed and how you will get them to relax in the interview also require consideration. Where the interview will actually be held is another crucial planning point. Again, this will depend on the nature of the interview. If undertaking a closed or semi-structured interview that is not covering very personal issues it may be acceptable to complete the interview in a public place. For example, market researchers often complete closed interviews in the street. The researcher exploring people's views of health care may feel that it is not unreasonable to do this in a relatively public place, for example a quiet corner in a hospital ward, as long as the conversation is not overheard. Interviews on more personal issues should always be conducted in a very private location.

ACTIVITY 20   ALLOW 5 MINUTES

Imagine you are planning to conduct an interview to ask colleagues what they feel about studying research through open learning methods. As far as you can determine, very little research has been done so far on assessing the use of open learning methods to help people learn about research. Answer the following questions.

1   Who will you interview?

2   Will you use a structured, semi-structured or open-interview approach?

3   How will you structure the questions in your interview schedule?

4   How will you collect the information? Will you write it down or use a tape recorder?

5   Where will you interview the interviewees and what will you need to consider before meeting them?

6   Are there any sensitive areas that might arise which could cause concern to an ethical committee?

Commentary

1   Obviously for this particular study you would need to interview people who have had some experience of open learning – otherwise they would not be able to answer your questions on this subject.

2   This kind of study would probably lend itself to a semi-structured approach and a framework for focused questions of the type shown below.

3   The kind of questions you might ask could be:

   ● why might open learning be preferred over other methods of learning?

   ● how is open learning study organised?

   ● what are the apparent strengths of open learning?

   ● what are the weaknesses?

4   It may be possible to write down the responses to such questions as they are likely to generate a fairly limited response. You could, of course, use a tape recorder but this might be felt to be more intimidating by the respondents.

5 It may be possible to meet people in a private area within a college or place of work. You will need to consider the importance of good interpersonal skills and the part they play in successful interviewing.

6 We would not expect any major ethical problems to arise in a study such as this, although that does not mean you should not be sensitive to potential individual sensitivities. For example, some people choosing open learning might be trying to make up for lost time on other programmes and have some additional pressure placed upon them to complete the course. They might therefore be unable to spend much time talking to you.

Conducting interviews

In conducting the interview you implement the plan of action you developed in the planning stage. A clear plan and care taken in implementing that plan are both important to the success of your interview. A few practical tips linked with interviews can usefully be adhered to. Remember that the communication skills required to conduct a research interview are the same as those used in any other kind of professional interview. You probably use such skills regularly without necessarily thinking about it. Be aware of the importance of body language and eye contact.

Remember that although people may know why you want to interview them a recap will help to 'set the scene'. Moreover, this will give you an opportunity to tell interviewees how you are going to conduct the interview, and, if you have not already done so, to tell them how you are going to record their responses. A statement such as 'I will be taking notes as we go through' will help them understand what you are doing. It is important not to take anything for granted in this situation, as it is quite possible that the people being interviewed may be nervous.

If you are intending to use a tape recorder you need to ask for permission to do so, even if you have already noted in an information letter that you will be using one. People do get nervous about being recorded. This may simply be owing to embarrassment about hearing themselves on tape or because they are concerned about who will hear the information. It is therefore both courteous and sensible to make sure that your interviewee knows exactly what you are going to do, both in recording data and what you will do with it once you have got it.

Reassurances about the confidential nature of the information gathered are essential. People usually forget that they are being recorded shortly after the process has started, so a few minutes' recording to get over nervousness will help. It will also give you an opportunity to check the practicalities of using a tape recorder, such as whether it is switched on, whether there is a tape in the machine, and the best position for recording both your own and your interviewee's voice.

ACTIVITY 21   ALLOW 15 MINUTES

Read the following scenarios which describe two different interview situations. Then:

1 List the differences between them under the headings 'Planning', 'Time keeping', 'Preparing equipment' and 'Establishing a rapport'.

2 Consider the impact these differences might have on the research data collected.

Marie is going to conduct a series of interviews for her research study into nurses' attitudes to the extension of their role into jobs previously carried out by medical staff. She hasn't spent much time planning her project and when she arrives at the first interview she hasn't given much thought as to how she will manage the situation. She is in a flustered state when she arrives and spends the first few minutes apologising as she tries to find her semi-structured interview schedule, which she has pushed to the bottom of her bag. She has forgotten to phone her interviewee, a staff nurse called Jo, to notify her of her impending arrival (although she had previously said she would do this). Therefore Jo is also quite flustered, because she is thinking of all the things she needs to do in the ward area. Marie spends a lot of time fiddling with the tape recorder – only to find that her tape does not work! Jo, in the meantime, is looking anxiously at her watch thinking of all the work she has to get through before lunch.

Eventually the interview begins and Marie starts to ask Jo questions. However, because she has to keep looking at her notes she does not establish good eye contact with Jo. As a result, Jo feels that Marie is not really interested in her answers and decides that the quickest way to get through the interview is to answer as briefly as possible. Jo feels quite nervous about what Marie is going to do with the information from the interview, as she has not been offered any confidentiality. Because Jo fears that Marie might tell her manager what she says, she is very guarded with her answers.

Lynn is going to conduct a series of interviews for her research study on nurses' views of trust status in the new NHS. She has spent a lot of time planning her projects and when she arrives at the first interview she has already given plenty of thought to how she will manage the situation.

She arrives at the meeting with her first interviewee in plenty of time. She gets her papers in order and puts her interview schedule on top of her pile of papers. She spends time setting up her tape recorder and testing it to make sure it works properly in the room set aside for this interview.

The person Lynn is going to interview is a staff nurse called Thomas. When she first contacted Thomas and asked him if he would be willing to be interviewed he indicated his willingness, but expressed reservations about variable workload on the wards that might influence his availability. Lynn told Thomas that she would telephone him on the day of the interview to see if it was still convenient to proceed. Thomas was therefore able to allow time for the interview and feels he has some control over the situation.

When the interview begins Lynn establishes a good rapport with Thomas by spending some time setting the scene, emphasising the confidential nature of the interview and assuring Thomas that, although the interview is being recorded, these data will only be available to her as the researcher. They also have a test-run to ensure that the tape will record the data correctly. Some laughter ensued as a result of this, which relaxed them both. Throughout the interview Thomas felt that Lynn was really interested in his ideas and felt inspired to share as many thoughts as possible with her. He viewed it as an opportunity to get his opinions heard.

Commentary

1   The differences you have listed between the two scenarios are probably to do with the degree of planning each researcher carried out, as shown in *Table 7* below.

	Marie	Lynn
Planning	Did not spend much time	Took time with planning
Time-keeping	Did not allow enough time	Allowed plenty of time
Preparing equipment	Did not do this adequately	Made an effort to ensure this was in working order
Establishing a rapport	Failed in initial promise to contact Jo and was too rushed to do this well	Kept promise to Thomas that she would contact him before interview and had time to explain

Table 7: The differences between Marie and Lynn's scenarios.

2   The data gathered by Marie were scantier than Lynn's because Jo felt less relaxed than Thomas. Marie's data would not be very accurate because Jo was being guarded in her responses. The information that Marie and Lynn had available to them after their interviews would be very different. Marie would probably have very little of use, while Lynn would have a great deal of insight into the subject.

The analysis stage

The analysis, or 'post interview' stage, could be said to begin with the closure of the interview – the point at which the interviewer thanks the person interviewed for his or her help. The researcher must now consider a number of issues. For example:

- will they need to do a follow-up interview?

- will they be sending the respondents a copy of the analysed data for verification?

- will they be sending respondents a copy of the completed research?

- are there any ethical issues that require follow up?

All of these issues will be very specific to each individual project and, in some cases to individuals within the project. Once they have been addressed the interviewer can begin the process of analysis. As noted, the way in which we collect data can be highly structured or semi- or low-structured. Highly structured data lend themselves to numerical forms of analysis, using either **descriptive** or **inferential statistics** depending on the orientation of the study (see Clifford and Harkin, 1997). **Content analysis** is the name given to the process of analysing data which is in the form of words rather than figures.

Broadly speaking, what the researcher has to do at this stage is to *transcribe* the information they have gathered into a format suitable for analysis. This means that if the interview data were collected by written response, the interviewer should return to the notes made in the interview as soon as possible on completion to make sure that the information is complete and accurate. If you have ever tried taking notes when someone is talking you will realise that it is not always possible to write out in full all the words that are said. This type of interview data needs to be checked and clarified as soon as possible after the interview; in other words, written out in full.

If the interview was tape recorded it is possible to leave it a little longer before transcribing the data in full, but an experienced researcher would probably suggest you do this before the next interview. There may be points raised that need clarifying, or issues raised that it may be useful to follow up in the next interview.

We will be considering the process of analysis for qualitative research in more detail in Session Four.

Descriptive statistics: *a type of statistics used to describe and summarise data effect. For example, the data from a research study may be presented in percentages as a means of summarising large sets of data.*

Inferential statistics: *a procedure in which statistical tests are used to infer whether the observations in the sample studied are likely to occur in a larger population.*

Content analysis: *the process of analysing data using words rather than figures.*

ACTIVITY 22   ALLOW 2 HOURS

Imagine you have been asked to act as a researcher in a study designed to gather people's views about the increase in homelessness in 1990s Britain. *Figure 3* gives three questions which form your semi-structured interview schedule. Spend about 15 minutes using this questionnaire with each of four friends or colleagues.

Before you start consider the following points.

● How will you choose your interviewees?

● Where will you arrange to meet them?

● How will you record the information you collect?

● Are there any special features to this research that you need to consider?

| 1   What are your views about homelessness? |
| 2   Do you feel that as individuals we should be doing anything about this? |
| 3   What do you feel society should be doing about this? |

Figure 3: Questions for use in homelessness questionnaire.

Commentary

We will be returning to the specific responses to your questionnaires in the next session. For the moment we want to examine how easy it was for you to work through the various stages in research interviewing.

1   Was it easy to identify people to help with your research? As you were using friends and/or colleagues you were probably able to choose people who might be helpful. This is not always the case in research projects, where you cannot rely on knowing the persons to be interviewed.

2   Where did you arrange to meet your interviewees and was this an easy or difficult thing to do? Did it feel a little contrived or was it something you felt you were doing naturally? Were you able to get access to a quiet office or corner of a room where you would not be disturbed, or did this turn out to be a difficult task? Again, this can sometimes be quite difficult to do in real life situations, where office space is short and quiet corners hard to find.

3   How easy did you find it to record the information? You probably found it too hard to keep up a conversation and write at the same time. You may not have been able to record all the detail you wanted. If you did it by using a tape recorder were you or your interviewee nervous of recording your voice on tape? If so, how did you overcome that?

4   Were there any special features of this research that you needed to consider? It is possible that the people you chose to ask about this particular subject may have given very little thought to the subject of homelessness and so found it difficult to respond to the questions asked.

✳ Focus group interviews

So far we have focused on one-to-one interviews, where the interviewer works with a single interviewee or respondent. Another approach that can be adopted to getting interview information involves asking a group of people what they feel about a particular situation. Known as a **focus group interview**, a group of 8-12 people is usually considered sufficient for this approach. For example, a researcher examining support services for people caring for elderly relatives or friends may decide to attend a local support group of carers and to ask them what they think of the services available.

The word 'focus' gives us a clue about the structure of the interview. The interviewer's task is to focus the attention of the group on one specific area. Thus it can be understood as a kind of semi-structured interview. Once focused on that area, the subject can be explored using semi-structured questionnaires. The emphasis is on semi-structured interviews because a highly structured approach

Focus group interview:
an interview technique in which a group of individuals are interviewed simultaneously.

would not work with a group. It would be hard to identify who responded to which question. Similarly, an open-question (low-structured) approach would make it very difficult to get to the heart of the matter in a group of people.

ACTIVITY 23
ALLOW 10 MINUTES

1 What do you think the advantages of a group interview might be?

2 What might the disadvantages of this approach be ?

Commentary

1 One advantage of a group interview is that the research can be done relatively cheaply and quickly. Interviewing several people at once can save time: for example, if there were ten people in a focus group interview lasting one hour, the same time for one-to-one interviews would be ten hours. Another advantage is that the researcher is able to explore topics more fully than is possible in one-to-one situations. People in group situations will stimulate alternative thoughts in each other. They will provide data from their group interaction (Morgan, 1993).

2 One major disadvantage of this approach lies in the high degree of skill in group management required of the researcher. This approach should not, therefore, be seen as an easy way to gather a lot of views.

Another difficulty lies in the way in which the data are recorded. If it is difficult to make notes and keep a conversation going in one-to-one interviews, imagine how much more difficult it is in a group setting. One way researchers overcome this is to involve two researchers in the interview, one to lead the interview and another to take responsibility for recording the data. It is possible to record a group interview on tape but you need to be sure that the equipment used is sensitive enough to pick up several voices.

Interviews are a very useful means of gathering data and can enable people to expand on their views and address issues in some depth. However, a potential weakness with the interview approach is that people may tell you what they think you want to hear and the way they actually react in a given situation may be different from the way they say they would react. In some research, therefore, particularly ethnographic, the researcher may want to see what *actually happens* rather than rely solely on what people say. This is called **observation**. We will now consider how this is used as a technique in data collection in research.

Observation:
a research method in which a researcher observes subjects in order to gather data. Observation research comprises both 'participation' and 'non-participation' research methods. The participant observer observes the subjects from within by becoming a member of the group he or she is researching. The non-participant observer observes the subjects from without by observing the group in his or her role as a researcher.

3: Using observation in qualitative research

Observation is a research method in which a researcher observes subjects in order to gather data. Observation techniques comprise both 'participation' and 'non-participation' approaches. The researcher using a non-participation approach will simply stand aside from the situation being observed and monitor what goes on. So, for example, a researcher observing how people in a multi-disciplinary team work together in hospital units will simply observe the team's activity without participating in any of the interactions. If the researcher were to join in any of the interactions he or she could actually change the group dynamics and this would have an impact on the data. In contrast to this, the participant-observer does join in the group activities and in effect becomes a member of the group he or she is researching. For example, a researcher undertaking an ethnographic study of how workers in a social work team manage their work might work so closely with social workers that, on occasion, he or she might help to manage specific problems under the supervision of the social worker.

Many of the principles of research design discussed in relation to using interviews in research apply to the use of observation. In the same way as interviews, observation can be carried out in a structured or an unstructured way and, again, needs to follow the same three processes of:

- planning the research

- conducting the research

- analysis of the data.

The planning stage in observation research is similar to that used in other forms of data collection. The first step is to decide whether this is actually the right approach for the study in question. Some studies clearly lend themselves more to observation than to interviews as the means of data collection. For example, if a researcher were going to examine how social workers used body language in their interviews with clients there would be little value in simply asking the social workers about this in an interview. The social worker would probably tell the researcher how he or she *thought* they used body language, which might not necessarily reflect what was actually done.

It is possible to observe in a very structured way or in an unstructured way, as illustrated in *Table 8*.

Highly structured	Semi-structured	Low-structured
Structured observation schedule	Focused areas of observation	Open observations
Fixed order/sequence of observing	Field notes used to record data	Field notes used to record data
Data can be analysed numerically	Data transcribed into words	Data transcribed into words

Table 8: Summary of approaches to observation.

Structured observation

As with an interview situation, if a researcher intended to do a highly structured observation study he or she would need to be very specific about the observations they were making. For example, if the researcher wished to observe how care assistants work he or she would not want to observe how the portering staff do their work. A structured observation implies a rigid *focus* to data collection. In other words, the researcher must have very clear categories of data to collect. So, in a care assistant study a researcher undertaking a structured observation approach would observe specifically what tasks the care assistants do and how long it takes them to do them.

To undertake a structured observation study then, the researcher must start with some pre-determined categories. Imagine that the owner of a department store wanted to find out what type of clientele used the store most. He asks a researcher to observe the range of people coming into the store. Several categories could be predetermined for the researcher, such as:

- young men

- young women

- middle-aged men

- middle-aged women

- elderly men

- elderly women.

As you have probably realised, this is a very crude list and would present some problems. For example, how would the researcher determine what age category people fit into? It might be easy to distinguish a young man or woman from an elderly man or woman but it is not so easy to distinguish between a young and a middle-aged man. This difficulty illustrates the need to be very specific about the categories that are being observed.

ACTIVITY 24   ALLOW 30 MINUTES

Identify a busy spot in a town centre – perhaps a railway station or a bus station – where you can sit unobtrusively for about 20 minutes and watch people passing by.

Take a copy of the checklist identified in *Table 9*. Place a tick in each column by the relevant description every time you observe somebody with a certain hair colour and degree of hair thinning. Only tick once for each person – don't tick twice if you see the same person twice. However, if you see someone with brown hair who is particularly bald, tick both categories in one column

People with:																
Brown hair																
Black hair																
Blond hair																
Red hair																
Grey hair																
Partially bald																
Completely bald																
Don't know (head covered)																

Table 9: Observation check list.

Commentary

This is quite a useful learning experience because it serves to demonstrate one of the difficulties in observation research – knowing exactly what you are supposed to be focusing on. For example, did you record each person's hair colour only once or do you think you may have indicated the same person on more than one occasion? How useful was the checklist in helping to focus your observations? Were there any categories of hair colour not identified? Refining your checklist is an important process in developing observation tools.

Semi–structured observation

Just as researchers can use semi-structured interviews, so they can use semi-structured observations, focusing on an area of interest in a rather more open way and asking what happens in situation X. In observing the situation, researchers will set some parameters but will not be so prescriptive as they would be in a structured observation.

For example, a researcher might use this approach if undertaking a study to monitor the nutritional state of people in hospital. To do this study he or she might decide to watch what happens at meal times and to focus the study around several areas, namely who gives out the food, who checks whether the patient has eaten it and who takes away the leftovers. In this situation the researcher would take notes centering around the categories noted. These notes are known as **field notes**. This name is used because the notes are taken in the 'field' – the term commonly used by qualitative researchers to indicate that the location of the research is a natural setting rather than the contrived setting of the laboratory.

Field notes: *the notes kept by a researcher undertaking an observation study 'in the field', a natural setting rather than a laboratory.*

Unstructured observation

This is the type of observation that is used in an 'open' observation study. In Session One we looked at a case study where Claire, a health worker going to a foreign country, wanted to find out as much as possible about the place. In that situation it was important for Claire to become involved in the situation and to be able to observe and sense what was happening around her.

The art of collecting data in an unstructured observation study, which largely consists of taking notes, can be quite a difficult one to master. As with the semi-structured approach, notes taken in this setting are called field notes. This approach is akin to the unstructured interview discussed above, in which a conversational approach is adopted. Here, however, the notes are derived from what is seen by the researcher in more general terms, rather like the researcher having a conversation with his or her own note book. This process is not as easy as it sounds. Focusing on specific areas for note taking can be quite difficult and the researcher must be able to keep the notes up to date. This, in turn, depends upon the nature of the observation. For example, the researcher who is completing a non-participant observation study can concentrate fully on what is happening around him or her and so can keep a fairly regular pattern in note taking. However, the researcher who is acting in a participatory capacity may have less time to keep notes up to date.

ACTIVITY 25   ALLOW 30 MINUTES

Next time you are sitting in a restaurant or café on your own, try and capture the experience of undertaking some unstructured observation. Imagine you are trying to study the culture of the waiter or waitress in order to understand his or her world through an observation study. Write down observations about what the waiters and waitresses do and the impact of this on the customers.

Commentary

You will have had different experiences in completing this exercise depending on the nature of the restaurant and the time of day you chose to complete the exercise. If you went into the restaurant at a fairly quiet time you may have noted that there were a limited number of waiters and waitresses available and that they were able to give their whole attention to customers as they served them. If, however, you went at a busy time you may have noted the pace at which they were working and the effect this had on the amount of time they could allocate to individual customers. Regardless of what you observed, the point of this exercise was to get you to experience the potential problems faced by an observer using an unstructured approach to observation. From an ethical perspective you could consider what the waiters and waitresses might feel if they knew you were watching them with a specific purpose, especially if you saw any aspects of poor practice.

Observational studies are likely to stir up more sensitivities than other forms of data collection and may, therefore, create more ethical problems. If someone is watching you at work there is a real risk that this could influence the way you approach your work.

ACTIVITY 26   ALLOW 2 MINUTES

Imagine a situation in which a researcher was coming to watch you and your colleagues in your work in order to study how health and social workers function and deal with their clients.

What factors about being observed might cause concern to you as an individual?

Commentary

You might be concerned because:

- you feel someone will be watching you to see whether you do something 'wrong'

- you fear you won't perform as well as your colleagues who are also being observed

- you fear that the researcher might be a 'spy' who will report your activities to your manager

- you are worried that the researcher might interfere with your work.

There is evidence from some observation studies that people do change their behaviour when they are being observed. This phenomenon is known as the **Hawthorn effect**, as it was first observed in an observation study in a factory of this name. The way researchers completing observation studies avoid this is to spend a period of time orientating themselves. Just as researchers carrying out interviews will spend some time getting to know the person being interviewed in order to put them at ease, in observational research researchers will spend time in the situation under study before starting to collect data. This has two advantages. First it allows the researcher to check out the proposed observational approach. Second, it allows the people being observed to relax in the presence of the researcher.

4: Using records in qualitative research

A third source of data used in qualitative research design is other documented records. For example, where researchers exploring the history of a profession will obviously not have direct access to early practitioners of the profession (who have long since died), they do have access to records and can use these to piece together fragments of those lives. These records might include diaries, medical records and letters. Similarly, records relating to existing situations can be used in research. Since in ethnography we use multiple sources of data to enable us to build a picture of the culture we are studying, records can be a very useful focus to help us in this process. Some of this data may be in numerical form, for example, population distributions. Much of it, however, will be in written form and so can be subjected to content analysis.

ACTIVITY 27   ALLOW 5 MINUTES

What type of records would health and social care practitioners be likely to have access to for use in a research project?

Commentary

Most practitioners would probably have access to care records of clients or patients. They might also find useful information in the archives of specialist clinical libraries.

Summary

1   In this session we have considered the collection of data in qualitative research design.

2   We have looked at the use of interviews and how these may be structured depending on the design of the research.

3   We have discussed the conduct of interviews and the importance of good interpersonal skills on the part of the researcher and used case studies as a means of illustrating these skills.

4   The planning and use of observation techniques has been explored and the use of records in qualitative research examined.

Before you move on to Session Four you should check that you have achieved the objectives given at the beginning of this session and, if not, review the appropriate sections.

SESSION FOUR

Analysing qualitative data

Introduction

In this session we will consider ways in which we can analyse qualitative data. We will be exploring content analysis in more detail and using worked examples to help you understand this process.

Session objectives

When you have completed this session you should be able to:

- describe how data collected in qualitative studies can be broken down into data display, reduction and interpretation

- explain how to undertake content analysis

- report findings from qualitative research

- recognise how to analyse data in different approaches to qualitative research.

1: Dealing with large volumes of data

The *volume* of data generated by different approaches to qualitative research can vary considerably. For example, if you collect qualitative data using a semi-structured questionnaire which asks respondents to reply to an open-ended question in six lines of space, you will be able to limit the number of words on the page. However, verbal responses to the same questions recorded on a tape recorder could be much more extensive. Researchers need to consider this matter when designing their studies.

Whatever the length of the response, the data will be subject to the same principles of analysis. However, the amount of information will influence the extent to which the analysis can be developed. The challenge to the researcher is to analyse the data in such a way that the findings from the study can be presented in a concise and logical way.

Miles and Hubermans (1994) argue that qualitative data analysis involves three stages:

- data display

- data reduction

- data interpretation.

We will use this framework to guide us through this session.

2: Data display

Once data have been collected they need to be organised or 'displayed' in a form that is accessible. The amount of time it takes to display the data depends to a large extent on the amount of data collected. For example, as indicated above, hand-written responses are likely to be shorter than tape recorded responses and will produce less data to display. Whatever the means used to collect the data, the first step in analysing them is to transcribe the responses in full.

ACTIVITY 28   ALLOW **60** MINUTES

Take one of the interviews about homelessness which you completed with a friend or colleague in Activity 22. Transcribe this interview in full, either writing it out in longhand or using a computer or typewriter if you have one. See how far you can get in the sixty minutes allocated to this activity.

Commentary

> You probably found this quite a laborious process. Unfortunately transcribing interviews, while tedious, is a necessary part of the research process in qualitative research. Of course, if you were actually undertaking a real life research project you would be spending a great deal longer displaying your data as you would have a larger number of interviews. You will understand now why it is a good idea to transcribe as you go along rather than leaving it all to the end of the research. Although we can use computers to help us in our analysis, we do not yet have an easy way of loading the data from interviews into computers without actually typing it in. Voice recognition computers may eventually be able to help with this task.

Having transcribed your interview you have completed the first step of data analysis in qualitative research: you have displayed your data in a visual form which enables you to look at it in more detail.

3: Data reduction

Once the data have been displayed, the next task is to reduce them to smaller units so that any trends or patterns can be identified (Miles and Hubermans, 1994). This process of content analysis is, again, quite time consuming.

Content analysis

One way of understanding how content analysis works is to review several newspapers and consider how the same story has been reported in each, identifying the common features and what has been mentioned less frequently. Similarly, if you were to interview a number of people about their satisfaction with work, it is quite likely that the subject of pay would emerge as a common feature and would be identifiable in every interview.

Content analysis can be applied to all qualitative data, although the degree of complexity with which this is done varies depending on the range of data available. We will start by looking at the most simple form of content analysis and then move on to a more complex form.

Content analysis of an open-ended questionnaire

Imagine we were doing a study designed to find out what people who had completed this open learning programme thought of this approach to learning. We have decided to use a questionnaire which includes some open-ended questions designed to elicit the views of the respondent. One such question is 'What do you think about open learning as a method of learning?' To begin our process of content analysis we need to see how all of the respondents answered this question. Our starting point here is to *collate* the responses, in other words, to collect all the responses to the same question together. There are several ways of doing this, the easiest of which is to transfer all the responses on to a word processing file. This gives the flexibility to manipulate the data at a later stage.

In response to our question 'What do you think about open learning as a method of learning?' we might gather the range of responses shown in *Figure 4*.

1. If I had the choice again I would prefer not to use this approach as I realise that I do prefer to be taught, rather than be self-directing in my learning.

2. I like open learning because I can work at my own pace.

3. I prefer open learning because everything is contained in the text and I do not have to spend a lot of time searching for materials to help.

4. Whilst I recognise there are benefits to open learning I miss the classroom and regular contact with my colleagues.

5. I tried this approach before for another course and I found that it was a good way to get into a subject but I would prefer to have more direct contact with tutors as the work develops.

6. Open learning is a good way to learn.

7. It is a good way to learn but not for me – I prefer to meet my teacher on a weekly basis.

8. I do not like open learning.

9. Open learning may be okay for some but not for me.

10. I really like this approach – it gives me the flexibility I need with the family. I can study whenever I feel I have the time.

Figure 4: Responses to the question 'What do you think about open learning?'

Faced with this range of responses we now need to take the first step in content analysis. To do this we need to look for any similarities or differences in the range of responses noted. As we have only got one page of responses here we can look at these data quite quickly and in so doing begin to get a 'feel' for the data: in other words, we begin to interpret the *patterns* in the responses. For example, can we say that all respondents like open learning? Is there a long list of apparent benefits emerging in the data or is there a generally negative view of open learning?

ACTIVITY 29   ALLOW 10 MINUTES

Look again at the range of responses on *Figure 4*. Can you see any similarities or differences in the range of responses noted?

List your observations in the margin alongside the responses.

Commentary

Several respondents were very positive about the approach (respondent numbers 2,3,6,10). Some respondents were negative, stating that they do not like open learning (respondent numbers 1 and 8), whilst others tended to be negative whilst recognising others may like this approach (numbers 4, 7, 9). Respondent 5 made suggestions as to how the approach could be improved.

Using this way of looking at the data we can begin to identify categories in responses. Our first step of analysis might, therefore, look like that in *Figure 5*.

1. If I had the choice again I would prefer not to use this approach as I realise that I do prefer to be taught rather than be self-directing in my learning.	Negative
2. I like open learning because I can work at my own pace.	Positive
3. I prefer open learning because everything is contained in the text and I do not have to spend a lot of time searching for materials to help.	Positive
4. Whilst I recognise there are benefits to open learning I miss the classroom and regular contact with my colleagues.	Positive and negative
5. I tried this approach before for another course and I found that it was a good way to get into a subject but I would prefer to have more direct contact with tutors as the work develops.	Positive; idea for developing
6. Open learning is a good way to learn.	Positive
7. It is a good way to learn but not for me – I prefer to meet my teacher on a weekly basis.	Positive and negative
8. I do not like open learning.	Negative
9. Open learning may be okay for some but not for me.	Positive and negative
10. I really like this approach – it gives me the flexibility I need with the family. I can study whenever I feel I have the time.	Positive

Figure 5: First stage in content analysis of questionnaire responses.

Looking at these statements in this way we can see that it is possible to identify those that have a fully positive orientation, those that have a negative orientation and those that are mixed. As we are dealing with a relatively small number of responses here we can state without too much difficulty that four respondents felt positively about open learning, whilst three respondents responded negatively and others held mixed views. We could present this data quite concisely by summarising it in one paragraph which states:

Four respondents were very positive about open learning whilst two were negative, stating they do not like it. Three others tended to be negative whilst recognising others may like this approach and one respondent (5) made suggestions as to how the approach could be developed.

Alternatively, we could present the summary in tabular form giving the full quotes as presented by the respondents (*Figure 6*).

Positive comments	Negative comments	Mixed
I like open learning because I can work at my own pace. Open learning is a good way to learn.	If I had the choice again I would prefer not to use this approach as I realise that I do prefer to be taught rather than be self-directing in my learning.	Whilst I recognise there are benefits to open learning I miss the classroom and regular contact with my colleagues.
I prefer open learning because everything is contained in the text and I do not have to spend a lot of time searching for materials to help.	I do not like open learning. Open learning may be okay for some but not for me.	I tried this approach before for another course and I found that it was a good way to get into a subject but I would prefer to have more direct contact with tutors as the work develops.
I really like this approach. It gives me the flexibility I need with the family. I can study whenever I feel I have the time.		It is a good way to learn but not for me – I prefer to meet my teacher on a weekly basis.

Figure 6: Summary of data in open learning questionnaire.

This form of grouping responses can be very useful. Here, this simple level of content analysis has served to indicate a range of views held by this group about open learning. Identifying trends or themes like this is described as 'latent content analysis' (Field and Morse, 1996).

Up to now, content analysis has been very straightforward. We have taken the short responses given by the respondents and presented them in tabular form. This is easy to do if the responses are short and concise, as in our example. However, we need to consider what we would do if the responses were more detailed. For example, let us take the response of respondent 10 above.

I really like this approach – it gives me the flexibility I need with the family. I can study whenever I feel I have the time.

Let us imagine the respondent had elaborated on this and stated:

I really like this approach – it gives me the flexibility I need with the family. I can study whenever I feel I have the time. What I do is get up early in the morning and do two hours

*before I get the children up and then when I come home from
work, do a couple of hours then.*

In this situation the researcher undertaking content analysis would need to
consider how relevant all the extra detail is to the original question asked. This
was 'What do you think about open learning as a method of learning?' The
question did *not* ask respondents how they organised their open learning
experiences so, although these data may be useful for the researcher as an
indication of how open learning can be organised, they are not relevant to the
actual question asked. The researcher would therefore make the decision not to
include all of these data in the analysis.

In discussing data that is not relevant to the study, Field and Morse (1996)
describe them as 'dross'. Although this could be seen as a pejorative term, the
reason for using it is to help the researcher focus on the issue in hand. In our open
learning example we have used very simple responses to illustrate the concept of
content analysis. As we continue our journey through content analysis we will
come across data such as those resulting from interviews which will contain
many more words. Using the idea of 'dross' helps the researcher to note from the
start which data are and are not relevant to the study.

Content analysis of open-ended interview questions

Open-ended questions in questionnaires give limited room for a response. We will
now address content analysis when longer responses are gathered to a question. We
will be using a worked example to demonstrate the key points that you should
consider in this type of content analysis, but at each stage you should return to the
data you gathered in your interviews about homelessness in Activity 22 to check
the points made.

In the questionnaire about homelessness in Activity 22 you will recall that one of
the interview questions was 'Tell me what you think about homelessness'. In
Figure 7 you will see an example of the data display of a possible response to the
interview question.

Well I think it is a terrible thing that in the 1990s in a modern society we have
a problem such as this. I don't know though what we can do about it. I want to
do something but I do not know what. You are constantly reminded of the
problem when you go to town. They are always there asking for money. It is
difficult because you do not know if they really need it or whether they are in fact
doing quite well from begging. But if you have any caring qualities you cannot
ignore requests for help when you have so much yourself.

They say a lot of people choose to live on the streets – they prefer it – well I do
not believe that. I think that is an easy thing for the authorities to say – it lets
them off the hook. So really I guess the answer to your question is that I am not
sure what to think about homelessness. I feel that something should be done
but I feel powerless to do anything personally. I think the time has come for the
government to do something. It makes me feel very uncomfortable – I do not
know what to do.

Figure 7: Data display of a possible response to the interview question 'Tell me what
you think about homelessness'.

Data of this length can be quite time-consuming to analyse. In focusing on a single
question the respondent has covered several issues in his or her response. You will
also have all the other responses to the same question to deal with, which could

be as long or longer. The starting point for our analysis here is to consider the response in full to get a 'feel' for what the respondent is saying.

ACTIVITY 30   ALLOW 5 MINUTES

Think about the responses in *Figure 7*. Is there an adjective you can use to summarise that response?

Commentary

Probably the best adjective to describe this response would be 'uncertain'. The respondent feels that homelessness should not exist but he or she is not sure what can be done to help resolve it.

Once the researcher has a sense of what this respondent is saying, he or she must try to identify any patterns in the data in order to analyse it further. In order to do this he or she will need to:

● break the data down into component parts

● look for commonalities across the data.

Breaking data down into component parts begins the process of data reduction.

Breaking data into component parts

The first component interview data can be broken down into is sentence units. This can help to give some indication of the areas covered, as shown in *Figure 8* below, where we have broken down the responses shown in *Figure 7*. A computer makes it very much easier to manipulate data as this can be done very simply in all word-processing packages.

ACTIVITY 31   ALLOW 10 MINUTES

Look at the sentences in *Figure 8* and underline what you think might be key ideas in each sentence. For example if the sentence was, 'I like a really hot cup of tea', you might underline 'hot' and 'tea' – I like a really <u>hot</u> cup of <u>tea</u> as the core idea of the sentence.

Well I think it is a terrible thing that in the 1990s in a modern society we have a problem such as this.

I don't know though what we can do about it.

I want to do something but I do not know what.

You are constantly reminded of the problem when you go to town.

They are always there asking for money.

It is difficult because you do not know if they really need it or whether they are in fact doing quite well from begging.

But if you have any caring qualities you cannot ignore requests for help when you have so much yourself.

They say a lot of people choose to live on the streets – they prefer it – well I do not believe that.

I think that is an easy thing for the authorities to say – it lets them off the hook.

So really I guess the answer to your question is that I am not sure what to think about homelessness.

I feel that something should be done but I feel powerless to do anything personally.

I think the time has come for the government to do something.

It makes me feel very uncomfortable – I do not know what to do.

Figure 8: The first step in data reduction.

Commentary

In *Figure 9* you can see what we consider to be key ideas. Don't worry if you have underlined other words – we are still only at the beginning of this process and there are no clear rights and wrongs. We are not claiming that this respondent's ideas are typical; rather, we are simply interested in this respondent's particular view.

Well I think it is a terrible thing that in the 1990s in a modern society we have <u>a problem</u> such as this.

<u>I don't know</u> though what we can do about it.

I want to do something but <u>I do not know</u> what.

You are constantly reminded of the <u>problem</u> when you go to town.

They are always there <u>asking for money</u>.

It is difficult because you do not know if they really need it or whether they are in fact doing quite well from <u>begging</u>.

But if you have any <u>caring</u> qualities you <u>cannot ignore</u> requests for help when you have so much yourself.

They say a lot of <u>people choose</u> to live on the streets – they prefer it – well I do not believe that.

I think that is an easy thing for the <u>authorities</u> to say - it <u>lets them off the hook</u>.

So really I guess the answer to your question is that I am <u>not sure</u> what to think about homelessness.

I feel that something should be done but I feel <u>powerless</u> to do anything personally.

I think the time has come for the <u>government to do something</u>.

It makes me feel very <u>uncomfortable</u> – <u>I do not know</u> what to do.

Figure 9: The second step in data reduction.

We have now gone through the process of data display (transcribing the data) and the two steps of data reduction (identifying key ideas from our data). In *Figure 9* we highlighted the following key words:

- problem
- do not know
- asking for money
- begging
- caring
- cannot ignore
- people choose
- authorities
- lets them off the hook
- not sure
- powerless
- government to do something
- uncomfortable.

This is quite a long list of words or concepts relating to the idea of homelessness. What we now need to do is reduce our data to smaller, more manageable units, by linking our words together to see if we can find patterns in the data. Frequency of occurrence of words and similarities in ideas will help us in this. This is the first step in data *interpretation*. Some words appear on several occasions and other words can be considered to have common meanings, for example, 'authorities' and 'government' fit together as a notion of control. Similarly, 'asking for money' can be linked with 'begging' in this case.

4: Data interpretation

We begin to interpret data by grouping words and ideas arising out of them in some logical way. You might list all those words that have a common association as shown in *Figure 10*. (We have not as yet given any headings to the categories in these figures as we will be returning to this point shortly.)

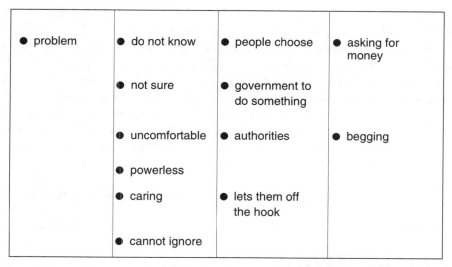

Figure 10: Common associations of the words in a response about homelessness.

You will note that the word 'problem' is on its own. That is quite acceptable because this is only the first interview and not a definitive model of the categories we will eventually be left with. We can anticipate that other words and ideas will emerge from other interviews as the work progresses.

Alternatively, you might draw a concept map on which you draw links between the words and ideas in your data, as in *Figure 11*.

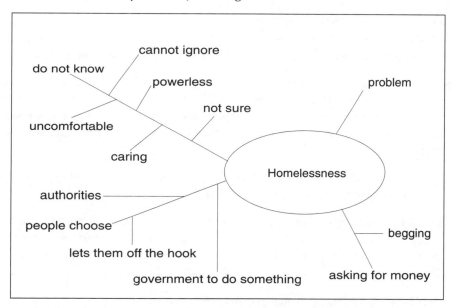

Figure 11: A concept map of the words used in a response about homelessness.

When we try to make these kinds of links some ideas fit together very easily, for example, words and ideas such as 'asking for money' and 'begging', or 'government' with 'authorities'. Other words do not fit together so neatly but may do so by association; for example, we might suggest that 'feeling uncomfortable' is due to 'uncertainty' or 'powerlessness'. You should not worry too much whether this is right or wrong at this stage because what you are doing is 'offering your interpretation' of these data.

To begin the process of data interpretation then, (the third stage of our data analysis) we need to look at our reduced data and try to 'develop themes', suggesting what they mean to us. So, for example, in *Figure 12*, the single word *problem* can stand alone as a heading to cover the idea of homelessness as a problem. The second group of data is formed by the words that indicate the *uncertainty* that the individual respondent experiences over this problem of homelessness. The third category, *delegation*, clearly links those issues relating to who should take responsibility for the problem. Is it the individuals' own choice to be homeless and therefore his or her own responsibility, or is it the responsibility of the government or the authorities? Both of these suggest that the problem needs to be delegated to someone. The final category shows the idea that when people ask for money they are begging and that these are a kind of *survival strategy*. By identifying themes in the data and indicating associations between them the process of *interpreting* the data from the interview has begun.

Problem	Uncertainty	Delegation	Survival tactics
● problem	● do not know	● people choose	● asking for money
	● not sure	● government to do something	
	● uncomfortable	● authorities	● begging
	● powerless		
	● caring	● lets them off the hook	
	● cannot ignore		

Figure 12: Data interpretation of responses – identifying categories.

These themes can also be inserted alongside the original data, as shown in *Figure 13*. This means that with a single set of data such as this we can extract quotes to illustrate where we are getting our interpretation from. For example, if we were trying to describe what was meant by uncertainty, we could illustrate it by the quotes:

> *I don't know though what we can do about it. I want to do something but I do not know what.*

This is useful when writing the report from this study but, more importantly at this stage of the analysis, it means that we have the data from one set of responses that can be grouped with another set of responses when looking for similarities.

Well I think it is a terrible thing that in the 1990s in a modern society we have a problem such as this.	Problem
I don't know though what we can do about it.	Uncertainty
I want to do something but I do not know what.	Uncertainty
You are constantly reminded of the problem when you go to town.	Problem
They are always there asking for money.	Survival tactics
It is difficult because you do not know if they really need it or whether they are in fact doing quite well from begging.	Survival tactics
But if you have any caring qualities you cannot ignore requests for help when you have so much yourself.	Uncertainty
They say a lot of people choose to live on the streets – they prefer it – well I do not believe that	Delegation

I think that is an easy thing for the _authorities_ to say – it _lets them off the hook_.	Delegation
So really I guess the answer to your question is that I am _not sure_ what to think about homelessness.	Uncertainty
I feel that something should be done but _I feel powerless_ to do anything personally.	Uncertainty
I think the time has come for the _government to do something_.	Delegation
It makes me feel very _uncomfortable_ – I _do not know_ what to do.	Uncertainty

Figure 13: Data interpretation.

Developing the themes

So far what we have done is simply to work through one short extract of interview data. When you are faced with the reality of doing your own qualitative research data analysis you will be dealing with a much larger volume of data. The stages we have outlined here might actually be developed on the basis of several complete sets of interview data. Whilst here we have been able to identify a small number of key words and ideas from a short extract of data, in your completed interviews you may be faced with 70 or 80 words or phrases that you wish to group in some way. This is where qualitative research analysis can become very cumbersome and shows why you need to keep careful note of each stage of the process as it develops.

ACTIVITY 32   ALLOW 30 MINUTES

Look at the second set of interview data about homelessness in *Figure 14*. Now analyse it by going through the stages described above:

1   Identify key words/ ideas in each sentence. How many of these are the same as the responses in *Figure 7*?

2   Do the ideas fit into the same categories as above? If not, can you identify any new categories?

3   Make an interpretation of Interviewee Two's views.

4   How does your interpretation of Interviewee Two's data differ from that of Interviewee One above?

I talked to some homeless people last year. They really changed my views about homelessness. They gave me a lot of reasons why it is better to live on the streets. Some of them said they did not like authority in society.

They said it could be uncomfortable but that they were able to get enough money by begging to buy odd luxuries like a hot cup of tea. It was interesting what they thought about begging for money. Some said they felt people were really embarrassed when they asked them for money – like it made them feel uncomfortable to be reminded that there were people without homes. However, they said others just looked at them with contempt – these they saw as the side of society they did not like – people in authority looking 'down their noses' at those who have less cash.

Mind you, I do not think this life would be the choice for all homeless people – there was one man whose wife had died and who had lost his job because he was so upset that he could not work. He had ended up on the streets when his house was repossessed. Talking to him made me feel very uncomfortable – I felt I should be able to do something to help.

Figure 14: Interviewee Two's response to the question 'Tell me what you think about homelessness'.

Commentary

A worked example of the breakdown of this interview can be found in *Figure 15* below. Although you probably found that some key words and ideas were the same as in the first interview, there are also some new ideas in the second interviewee's response. For example, the idea of people choosing to be homeless is emphasised in this interview as a positive feature of homelessness. The idea of authority is also introduced here, but from the perspective of some homeless people's contempt for authority. This interviewee also suggested that the homeless 'like to live on the streets;' there was some indication of that in the idea of 'delegation' in our first interview. Both interviewees felt uncomfortable about homelessness but the second interviewee empathised with the positive attitude of some people who want to live on the streets and appeared to have a different attitude because of the insights gained. Note that 'embarrassment' was recognised by the second interviewee but from the perspective of the person doing the giving, whereas with Interviewee One it was the people who were given money that were embarrassed.

In *Figure 16* we have put the categories that we identified above from Interviewee One and set the new categories from the second interview below that. You can see that we have some overlap in ideas relating to 'uncertainty' and 'survival tactics'. The new categories identified include 'insight,' 'homelessness as a preferred option', 'a rejection of authority' and 'embarrassment resulting from begging'.

I talked to some homeless people last year. They really changed my views about homelessness.	Insight
They gave me a lot of reasons why it is <u>better to live on the streets.</u>	Favoured option
Some of them said they <u>did not like authority</u> in society.	Dislike authority
They said it could be <u>uncomfortable</u> but that they were able to get enough money by <u>begging</u> to buy odd luxuries like a hot cup of tea.	Uncertainty Survival tactics
It was interesting what they thought about <u>begging</u> for money.	Survival tactics
Some said they felt people were really <u>embarrassed</u> when they asked them for money – like it made them feel <u>uncomfortable</u> to be reminded that there were people without homes.	Embarrassment Uncertainty
However, they said others just looked at them with <u>contempt</u> – these they saw as the side of society they did not like – people in <u>authority</u> looking 'down their noses' at those who have less cash.	Contempt Do not like authority
Mind you, I do not think this life would be the <u>choice for all</u> homeless people – there was one man whose wife had died and who had lost his job because he was so upset that he could not work. He had <u>ended up</u> on the streets when his house was reclaimed.	Lack of choice Lack of choice
Talking to him made me feel very <u>uncomfortable</u> – I felt I should be able to do something to help	Uncertainty

Figure 15: Analysis of Interviewee Two's response to the question 'Tell me what you think about homelessness'.

Interviewee One

Problem	Uncertainty	Delegation	Survival tactics
● problem	● do not know	● people choose	● asking for money
	● not sure		
	● uncomfortable	● government to do something	● begging
	● powerless	● authorities	
	● caring	● lets them off the hook	
	● cannot ignore		

Interviewee Two

Insight	Preferred option	Reject authority	Embarrassment
● insight	● better to live on the streets	● do not like ● uncomfortable in authority	● contempt from people

Figure 16: Categories from Interviewee One (see *Figure 12*) with additional categories from Interviewee Two.

Overall, this is how we gradually achieve data analysis in qualitative research. Each question is looked at in this way and, in breaking it down into component parts, our goal is to look for common meanings. If we were to continue the process of analysing responses to the same question that we have been using here, it is likely that we would find a similar pattern to that we have identified above. We might expect different responses, but within them find that some responses reflect those categories we have already identified. New categories would be added as we went along. Experienced qualitative researchers will advise you that the process of data collection and analysis continues until **saturation of categories** is reached; until we are no longer adding new categories to our data.

5: Analysing data in different approaches to qualitative research

Broadly speaking, the steps outlined above would be followed for the analysis of the data in descriptive, exploratory and interpretative approaches, but the interpretation of those data might vary. For example, if you were undertaking a descriptive/exploratory study you might categorise your data as described above and then present your report. However, if you had been undertaking this study as part of an ethnographic study into the culture of homelessness, you would want to challenge every aspect of those data from a cultural perspective. If you were a phenomenologist, you would probably be more concerned with how the individual feels about homelessness and what impact it has on them. If you were a grounded theorist your approach to data analysis might be very specific. You might use those data to propose theories related to people in general's perception of homelessness and develop further studies from that, for example, using the data to develop a questionnaire to ask a wider group of respondents their views of homelessness.

Summary

1   In this session we have considered the process of analysing qualitative data.

2   We have described how data collected in qualitative studies can be broken down into data display, reduction and interpretation.

3   We have considered content analysis of data and the various stages of achieving this.

4 We have seen that data interpretation can also be carried out through concept mapping and discussed how themes relevant to the research are identified through this technique.

Before you move on to Session Five you should check that you have achieved the objectives given at the beginning of this session and, if not, review the appropriate sections.

Reading and using qualitative design research reports

Introduction

In this session we focus on how to read and judge the quality of a qualitative design research report. This will help you to critically read and understand the implications of published qualitative research. It will also help you to identify situations in which qualitative research is used in practice.

Session objectives

When you have completed this session you should be able to:

- critically read a published research study that has used qualitative research design

- distinguish between research reports that have a descriptive /exploratory orientation and those with an interpretative orientation (either ethnographic, phenomenological or grounded theory)

- discuss how qualitative research can be used to influence practice and further development of knowledge.

1: Reading published research reports

Reading published research reports is usually described either as 'research review' or 'research critique'. Although these terms are used interchangeably, it should be noted that the review is often simply that: a review of the research literature in the field of study. A research critique, however, is more focused. It is undertaken in order to ascertain the merits of a piece of research. The skills required for undertaking a research critique are important for all health and social care professionals, since it is only by understanding the results of a research report that you will be able to decide whether the results actually have any use for you. You therefore need to be sure you have sufficient knowledge of the principles of qualitative research design to be able to undertake such a critique.

The process

The process of research critiquing demands a fairly good level of knowledge on which to base conclusions. Many research texts offer advice on how to critically read a research report and, in so doing, focus on the broad framework of the research process that we have covered so far in this text. This includes information such as:

- the purpose of the study

- any supporting literature leading to the overall research design

- any ethical issues that emerge in the study

- the findings and conclusion related to the stated purpose of the study.

Whatever the text you look at for advice on research critique you will find that, in general, the principles given are the same but that the degree of detail incorporated in the advice varies. The general points which need to be considered when reading research reports are listed in *Table 10* and we elaborate on these further below.

- The **title** of the report – is it concise and to the point?

- The **abstract** – is it focused and to the point?

Introduction

- Is the **purpose** of the research identified and the **significance** of the problem to professional practice stated?

- Is the related **literature** discussed?

Research design

- Is the research **design** clearly stated – is it appropriate to the subject under study?

- Are the **techniques of data collection** clearly identified?

- Is the **location** of the study noted?

- Is the **sample** identified and the means of involving participants indicated?

Ethical issues and access

- Are the ethical implications of the research noted?

- Has access to the research been negotiated?

Data analysis

- Is the process of analysing data spelt out?

- Is there any other information you might have required to understand this?

Findings/Conclusion

- Are the findings discussed and linked to the literature and existing theory if appropriate?

- Are there any suggestions for using the research?

- Are the implications for future research considered?

Overall style

- Is the paper easy to read and accessible to professional readers?

References

- Are these complete and up to date both in the text and in the references list?

Table 10: Issues to consider when critically reading research reports.

The **title** of the report needs to be concise as it is the title of the article which is used when research reports are indexed in libraries. The **abstract** is usually about 100-200 words and located at the beginning of the research report. Its purpose is to give a concise summary of the contents of the research report. If the abstract is a good representation of the contents of the article it can save you, the reader, a lot of time. It is often by reading the abstract that we decide whether or not the whole article has relevance for us.

The **purpose** of the research and its **significance** for practice should be clearly identified in the introduction. It should draw on existing literature to demonstrate the need to undertake the project and show why the research might be important for health and social workers. You will recall from Session Two, however, that the way researchers refer to the **literature** varies in different forms of qualitative research design. Traditional, quantitative approaches to research begin with a literature review in which all the related material is brought together at the outset. However, in a number of qualitative research reports, the literature will be drawn into the study as it progresses. So, for example, in a phenomenological study you would probably not see a discrete section labelled 'literature' but would see the literature integrated throughout and used to illustrate points as the report develops.

The next question to ask is whether the **research design** is clearly stated and appropriate to the subject being studied. For example, if we were to read a research report which claimed to be doing a phenomenological study but which was in fact doing an ethnographic study, the researcher might be challenged. Next, we ask whether the **techniques of data collection** are clearly identified. As we saw in Session Three, in qualitative research we expect data to be collected through questionnaires, interviews and observation. Each method has particular features to recommend it, as well as certain weaknesses. You would expect a research report to include recognition of the strengths and weaknesses of using the particular approach to data collection selected.

Whilst it would not be usual for the researcher to note the exact **location** of a research study for ethical reasons (for example, because of confidentiality) there should be some general indication of the location of the study to enable readers to detect any potential for bias or weakness in the research design. For example, if a researcher said she was going to do an ethnographic study of the culture in a hospital ward and then proceeded to describe the culture of a community care hostel we would challenge her perspective. The location of the interviews may influence the way in which the researcher and subject relate to each other, which in turn will influence the quality of the data collected. Consider, for example, a situation in which a probation officer is going to interview a number of young offenders. He decides to do so in the police station when the young offenders are awaiting a decision about their future. The probation officer might want to compare this interview with another one carried out a few weeks later in the offenders' homes. The interviewees' concern about impending prosecution at the later stage would probably be less acute than when they were first taken into custody and so they might be more willing to share more of their feelings.

The research report should indicate the size of the **sample** and the ways in which it was selected, following the principles of sample selection for qualitative research discussed in Session Two. We noted there that you would expect small samples in qualitative research studies, with selection being determined by the experiences the sample group has to offer the researcher. The samples would be described as purposive, theoretical or opportunistic. Some mention should be made of **ethics** in the research report, so that readers can be sure that good practice has been maintained.

The way in which **data are analysed** should be spelt out sufficiently to enable the reader to understand the thinking that went on behind each step of the process. In other words, the reader should be able to understand what was done. If the process was cumbersome the researcher may choose to summarise the process by making reference to another text. For example, the researcher might note that he or she followed the steps defined by Strauss and Corbin (1990). The reader would then need look up this approach in the text referred to.

It is vital that the critical reader should consider whether the **findings** clearly arise out of the research and whether they are discussed in an unbiased fashion by the researcher. It is very easy for researchers to slip into a biased perspective when reporting findings. Qualitative researchers are often undertaking research into areas where little is known of the subject and where there is little existing literature. It is particularly important in such situations to assess the researcher's possible bias.

Any **recommendations** arising out of the research and suggestions for using the research findings or for carrying out future research should, similarly, be critically assessed. **References** should be complete. Articles referred to in the text should be accurately presented at the end. References should also be 'up to date', although this is not an easy thing to define. For example, if a researcher is undertaking a qualitative research study in an area where very little research had been completed in the past, the only references available to them in the context of this study may date back many years. If, on reading an article on a subject you are familiar with, you see that a number of research papers published in the last couple of years have not been cited in the references, you might then question how complete and up to date those references are.

ACTIVITY 33   ALLOW 1 HOUR

Turn to *Resource 2* in the *Resources Section*, a paper on the psychosocial needs of patients who have attempted suicide by overdose. Read through the report once, critically, and then, on your own paper, write a few words under each heading from the list in *Table 10*.

Commentary

Now review your answer in the context of the comments below.

- The title of the report – is it concise and to the point ?

  Carrigan's paper is entitled 'The psychosocial needs of patients who have attempted suicide by overdose'. This is a very concise title that focuses on the nature of the research and the specific sample group. It is a good title for indexing purposes.

- The abstract – is this focused and to the point?

  The abstract for this paper is a very concise overview of the research that is reported beneath it. It identifies the research design, the sample selection, the method of data analysis, the findings and the conclusions.

Introduction

- Is the purpose of the research identified and the significance of the problem to professional practice stated ?

  The purpose of the research is clearly stated under the heading 'The study'. Carrigan states that the aim of the study is to 'investigate and highlight the psychosocial needs as perceived by individuals who have survived an attempt of deliberate self-poisoning'. This is a rather more complicated way of stating the same thing noted in the title, but the researcher wisely chose a neater and shorter title to summarise what the study was about.

  In this section Carrigan also notes that the research set out to evaluate health care support received during and following the incident. This could be confusing, as he does not clearly state that this support is in the realm of psychosocial support and suggests that another dimension not included in the title is being introduced into the study. Support for this aspect can also be seen in the literature review.

Literature

● Throughout the literature review, Carrigan endeavours to link the literature to the implications for nursing and so keeps the purpose of his study to the forefront. He has presented the literature initially in the traditional format, beginning the paper with an overview of the existing literature before going on to describe a number of theoretical perspectives that have relevance for the study. Overall it can be said that the section on the literature constitutes a review of relevant information rather than a *critique,* as there is limited evidence of the author critically analysing any of the papers referred to.

Carrigan returns to the literature later in the paper and also weaves his findings into the report itself, as we shall see in the section on data analysis below. However, at this point it is worth noting that although Carrigan states that the framework used for the analysis is drawn from themes in the literature, these particular themes are not developed in the results section, where other sources of literature, not previously referred to, appear.

Research design

● Is the research design clearly stated – is it relevant to the subject being studied?

The research design is clearly identified as an exploratory, descriptive design. This does appear relevant to the subject being studied because a study of such a sensitive nature would not lend itself to other approaches. For example, it would not be appropriate to circulate questionnaires to people in such a sensitive health state, asking them what their needs are. Neither would it be appropriate to undertake any observation work, since this would neither answer the question nor be ethically correct, again because of the sensitive nature of the problem.

● Are the techniques of data collection clearly identified?

Yes. Carrigan notes the use of 'focused' interviews, which could entail the use of a semi-structured interview schedule. Although the questions were prepared in advance the interviews were 'non-directive to a point, in that the order and content of the questions depended on the individual response'. This description fits with our earlier description of semi-structured interview schedules.

● Is the location of the study noted?

It was noted that initial contact was made in the hospital ward where this sample group were admitted after the overdose attempt. The actual research was completed in the respondents' own homes after discharge.

● Is the sample identified and the means of involving participants indicated?

It was clearly stated that there were three females and three males. This was cited as a 'sample of convenience', readily accessible to the researcher. In other words, this is an opportunistic sample. We can assume that this was a purposive sample, as the researcher selected people who suffered from the particular phenomenon under study. Carrigan does not actually state this.

Ethical issues

● Are the ethical implications of the research noted?

This is obviously a very sensitive area for study and Carrigan has made sure that the ethical issues are covered in his paper. He makes a clear statement about getting permission from the local ethical committee to undertake the study. It is also noted that verbal permission was sought from the sample group when the study was explained to them. Respondents were told how their names had been identified, although this is not clear to the reader. It was apparent that in arranging to meet this group once they had been discharged from the hospital, the researcher was addressing the ethical issues of attempting to interview people still in an acute state in hospital.

- Has access to the research been negotiated?

Permission for access was obtained from the appropriate consultant and nursing staff.

Data analysis

- Is the process of analysing data spelt out?

Is there any other information you might have required to understand this?

Carrigan includes a concise paragraph about the process involved in data analysis by making reference to a framework of 'latent' and 'manifest' analysis described by Field and Morse (1996). Reference to that text shows that 'latent analysis involves the review of sentences, passages and paragraphs to identify themes in the data, whilst manifest analysis focuses on words or phrases in the data that may emerge with sufficient frequency to be counted'. This enables the researcher to see how frequently specific themes emerge. So, for example, Carrigan noted that four respondents expressed feelings of poor self-esteem.

It is common at this stage for readers of qualitative research reports to find that they need to rely on the interpretation of the researcher. Since we do not have access to the original data to determine whether the selection of themes and ideas is appropriate, we can only *assume* that this has been done appropriately. The space available in journal articles does not allow the researcher to state any more than an overview.

Findings/conclusion

Carrigan notes that he used the themes that had emerged in the literature review to set the framework for his report of findings. Existing theory was clearly used, with reference to the use of developmental theories, stressful life events and social integration. Throughout the review of findings, Carrigan uses quotes from respondents to support the interpretation and draws on relevant literature to discuss the implications of this data.

Throughout the report Carrigan also raises issues of relevance to practice in highlighting issues that are relevant to care. He notes that the limitations of the study lie in the small number of people involved in the data collection and the varied length of time between the initial overdose and the research interview, which may have affected the data. He also notes that 'some' subjects refused to stay in hospital which may have meant they had different needs. However, he does not state how many 'some' represented. This raises issues about future research which Carrigan does not discuss. Carrigan has highlighted a number of issues in the framework of a qualitative research report, however this is an area which warrants future research. A broader understanding of the needs of this client group could clearly influence the care given to them.

Overall style

- Is the paper easy to read and accessible to professional readers?

The paper is logically presented and should be accessible to most practitioners with an interest in this field of practice.

References are complete and up to date, indicating a wide review of the literature.

The last activity involved critically reading a qualitative *descriptive* research design. Brockup and Hastings-Tholsma (1995) have noted the specific issues that would need to be considered when reviewing other approaches to qualitative research design. For example, they note that in an ethnographic study readers would need to check whether the researcher conducted the research in a practical setting and whether the researcher was involved in the data collection process as an observer, participant observer or interviewer.

In reading phenomenological research, these authors suggest questioning whether the researcher studied the phenomenon from the perspective of the participant. In the context of the grounded theory approach readers should ask 'Is the social situation under study clearly indicated by the researcher and does the researcher attempt to develop a theory about the social situation that is based on a combination of observation and literature review?'

2: Research in practice

You will recall from Session Two that when using *quantitative* research the researcher uses techniques of data collection and data analysis to enable them to undertake statistical tests to determine whether the results from his or her study could be generalised to the whole population. This contrasts with qualitative research, in which the study is focused on a much smaller sample and, on the search for meanings and insights into a given situation. We are therefore not generating data to apply to the wider population but are simply trying to increase our understanding by focusing on a smaller population. This can serve to clarify ideas on how we might approach situations in our own work.

ACTIVITY 34	ALLOW 10 MINUTES

Reflect on the article by Carrigan (Resource 2) and consider the areas of new awareness it brought up about caring for people who have attempted suicide.

Commentary

The kind of things you may have listed will depend largely on your own insight into the subject. There are no right and wrong answers, but you could have included:

- increased awareness about the nature of the problem

- questions about the statistics used – are the ratios of potential suicide the same in 1996 as they were in the literature cited on page 635 dating from 1987?

- a challenge to nurses to use the theoretical literature

- increased sensitivity to the impact of poor self-esteem

- increased sensitivity to the need of people to be loved and to have control

- questions about the issue headed 'the need to escape'

- limitations in the nursing response when trying to meet the needs of this group

- the need for follow-up support when patients are discharged from hospital

- the potential problems encountered in communicating within families.

As Carrigan noted, there are a number of limitations in the study but it has nonetheless served a purpose in increasing our sensitivity to the feelings of a particularly vulnerable group. We would not be allowed to rush out and change practice or procedures in a big way on the basis of such a small-scale study if we were hospital managers. However, in raising these issues and some potential solutions Carrigan is pointing a way forward for developing practice. Simply by highlighting the feelings of his group of respondents – for example, that nurses could have approached the care of this group in a more understanding way – Carrigan can help nurse managers to review the practices in their own situations.

It is quite possible that issues raised in qualitative research design will open up further questions for research that could be developed using a qualitative or quantitative approach – or by drawing on triangulation, as discussed earlier. Carrigan, for example, noted limitations in his study relating to the lack of representativeness of his sample, his own subjective interpretation of the study, the length of time between the overdose and the interview and the fact that some potential respondents did not wish to participate in the study. He rightly notes that despite its limitations the study raises some useful insights. If you were wanting to undertake your own study in this area you might pick up and develop a study to address some of the limitations noted.

Summary

1 In this session we considered how to read and use qualitative research reports.

2 We began by considering the necessary skills and knowledge required for reading published research reports.

3 We discussed the systematic process adopted for critical analysis. This was organised under headings that are transferable to most published research analysis.

Before you move on to Session Six you should check that you have achieved the objectives given at the beginning of this session and, if not, review the appropriate sections.

SESSION SIX

Writing a research proposal for qualitative design

Introduction

In this session we focus on writing for qualitative design. The purpose of this is to help plan a research study and write a research proposal for qualitative design. We briefly explore the principle of writing a research report after completion of a qualitative study.

Session objectives

When you have completed this session you should be able to:

- plan a research study using a qualitative approach

- write a research proposal for qualitative design.

1: Planning a research proposal

When we want to go on holiday we are unlikely to leave making our plans until the day before we go. We are more likely to make plans in advance. Similarly, before we undertake a research study we need to consider carefully what we want to achieve and where and how to achieve it. In research this process is known as writing a research proposal. A research proposal is simply a plan of action for a study.

ACTIVITY 35   ALLOW **10** MINUTES

Think about the potential benefits of writing a plan before you undertake a research project and list them below.

Commentary

The kind of things you might have written in your list are that a plan:

- helps to clarify exactly what you want to do

- gives a goal for the research

- sets out what you want to achieve and how you will achieve it

- gives you an opportunity to identify exactly why your proposed work is important.

The basic principles of writing a research proposal are the same regardless of the reason for writing it. However, you should note that if you have been asked to write a proposal by someone else – such as a teacher for an assignment on a research programme, or by a funding body for research – it is likely you will be given specific guidelines as to how this is to be done. For example, if doing an assignment it is the usual practice for a course tutor to provide some information about what to present and how to present it. This is commonly accompanied by a stated word limit that will give some focus to your work. In the same way, organisations that offer funds for research will give a framework for proposals and, again, commonly specify the maximum length. Funding bodies will specify how many pages proposals should be and will, again, put a limitation on the number of words used. If you are applying for funds for research you are advised to get some external advice from someone who is used to looking at proposals to examine the issues we raise here.

A research proposal generally covers a similar range of categories to those covered in the previous session in a research report. The difference is that a proposal is a statement of intent, whilst a research report is a statement of what has been done.

ACTIVITY 36 ALLOW **10** MINUTES

Note down the issues you should consider if you are planning a research proposal. Remember, a proposal is a statement of intent about what you intend to do and how you intend to do it.

Commentary

The kind of things you should have listed include:

- thinking about what you want to research – define your research question

- finding out whether any one else has undertaken this research before, perhaps by asking an expert (a supervisor or a teacher) or by searching the academic literature to see if you can find anything on the topic

- thinking about why the research you propose is important

- thinking about how you might research it – what approach would be appropriate for you to use and what research design would be appropriate

- considering how you might collect the data

- considering whether there are likely to be any ethical dilemmas in undertaking this work – for example, do you want to observe any sensitive situations

- how you might analyse the data

- how you would present the results.

2: Writing a research proposal in qualitative design

The starting point for any project is the stated aim of the project or the research question. The next step is to consider why this project is worthy of research. As this is not something we have covered so far it is worth considering here in a little more detail.

ACTIVITY 37 ALLOW **5** MINUTES

Read the scenario in the box below and consider why Vivienne's manager may not be too pleased about choice of topic.

Vivienne is a social worker undertaking a research course which entails spending one evening a week at college. Her employers have given her support to do this course. They have given the time for her to go to college, as well as some assistance towards the course costs. Her managers are hoping that the research project Vivienne will complete as part of her study will be useful for them and provide a return on their investment in her time for study.

When Vivienne is ready to undertake her project work she comes to her managers and states that she wants to explore people's attitudes to eating meat. When asked to justify why she has chosen this project she tells her manager that she feels very strongly about meat eating and she wants to understand what factors influence people's choice of diet. Her manager is not very pleased about this choice of topic and Vivienne does not understand why.

Commentary

Vivienne's idea for research is quite acceptable in general but the problem is the context in which she plans to do it. Since she has been supported by her managers in undertaking a research course, they obviously expect her work to reflect some area of need in their own environment of social work practice. In this case it is hard for Vivienne to justify why this research is important, as it does not link to her work in any way. If she were supporting herself to do her studies she might pursue a question which is of personal interest to her. Equally, if she were a dietician, it might be a valid area of study because, regardless of personal preference, it is important for a dietician to understand the factors that influence the diet people eat.

Now compare Viviene's situation to another scenario.

Ken is a health care worker who is interested in change processes in health care organisations. Over recent years the national policy has been to implement a new system in which care is delivered by NHS trusts. Ken feels that whilst some aspects of this change are positive for patient care other aspects may not be so good. He wants to undertake a study that will enable him to make recommendations for change in the NHS. He will do this work as part of a small research methods course and so has a limited time in which to complete it. Ken feels that as this is a new area about which little is known, it would be more appropriate to undertake a qualitative study. He intends to use a process of purposive sampling to interview ten colleagues. Ken's research question is: 'What do health care workers thinks of the new NHS?' He decides to collect the data using an open interview approach in a conversational style.

ACTIVITY 38   ALLOW 5 MINUTES

Write down any flaws you can see in the work Ken proposes to do.

Commentary

The major flaw in Ken's idea is that he is planning to make recommendations for change based on what is clearly a descriptive/exploratory study. Although he may well find that the people he interviews express strong opinions about the way the new NHS could be modified, he is not in a position to make recommendations for change as he has chosen to undertake a *qualitative* approach. Remember, the purpose of qualitative research is to unearth new knowledge or to present the idea at a descriptive level. If Ken simply said that he was using the study to identify NHS workers' views about the NHS this would be perfectly acceptable, as he would not be planning to make recommendations for change based on a small sample size in qualitative design.

Let us assume that, following discussion with her manager, Vivienne changes her topic to one that has practical significance to her work, such as finding out more about how the social work team function. She frames the question 'How does an inner city social work team function?'

Vivienne's manager has had some concerns about team dynamics over recent months and thinks that this is a well justified piece of work. Moreover, when Vivienne searches the literature to ensure that this topic has not been over researched in the past, she finds that it is an area in which very little work has been done. She decides that a qualitatively oriented study to explore or describe what is happening in the social work team would be the most suitable approach.

The contents of a research proposal

Vivienne is now ready to prepare her proposal and to do so will follow the broad steps outlined below in *Table 11*, which outlines the content of what to include in a research proposal. You will note that the broad framework of this table is similar to that of *Table 10* in Session Five, which indicated the areas you would review when reading a research report. The major difference is that when writing a research proposal you are writing in the *future tense*, since you are noting what you *intend* to do. In the research report we reviewed in the last session, Carrigan was writing about what he had *done*.

- Clear *title*

Introduction

- The purpose of the research is identified and the significance of the problem to professional practice stated
- Relevant *literature* is discussed

Research design

- Clear statement of research design
- Identify *techniques of data collection*
- Identify location of the study
- Identify the *sample*

Ethical issues and access to the research site

- Note any potential ethical dilemmas
- Access to the research is clarified

Data analysis

- State the way in which data will be analysed

Additional information including

- Time scales
- Project cost

Conclusion

- Have the implications and potential outcomes of the research been considered?

References

- Are these complete and up to date in the text and in the references list?

Overall style/presentation

- Is the proposal easy to read and accessible to both professional and non-professional readers?

Table 11: Framework for a research proposal.

In general, the basic principles of good writing apply just as much when preparing a research proposal as with any other writing:

- think carefully about what you are going to write under each heading

- plan what you are going to say

- think about sentence and paragraph construction

- be prepared to have someone read your work objectively when you have completed it.

A number of texts are available which cover writing skills for research (see, for example, Clifford and Gough, 1990). It would be a good idea to look through such a text before beginning to write.

We will now work through the headings in *Table 11*.

The title should be clear and concise and suitable for indexing purposes. If we use our example of Vivienne above, the title of the study might be: 'Social work in the inner city'. This clearly indicates the focus of the research in a specific group – social workers – and in a specific area – the inner city. The title could perhaps be extended to indicate the nature of the study, for example, 'Social work in the inner city: a qualitative research study'. However, care should be taken that it does not get too unwieldy.

The introduction is the first part of your proposal that will be read, so you need to ensure that it grasps your readers' attention. It should give an overview of what is to come and be presented in a concise and interesting way. It is very important that you state the aims of your work or the question that you are going to ask at the outset of your proposal, since all the work that follows will build upon the initial question that you ask.

Detailing the literature available which relates to your research topic is important, as it can serve to support your choice of study. You will need to consider how you might use the literature to support your perceived need for this particular research work to be done. For example, if you have searched the literature and found very little information about a chosen topic or found that the literature illustrates that a particular area has been reviewed in some depth but not from a *qualitative* angle, then your study will be shown to be necessary and justifiable.

The research design needs to flow logically from your stated research question, as it will determine the way in which you intend to carry out your research. At this point you will state clearly that the design will be qualitative, and describe the overall methodological approach you are going to take, whether ethnographic, phenomenological or using grounded theory. The important point here is that the way you design your study should be consistent with the questions you are asking. In Session Two, where we looked at differing research questions, we noted for example that the questions that began with 'what does it feel like to be...' were more suited to phenomenological research.

Techniques of data collection will be driven by the overall research design. For example, if Vivienne wanted to undertake an ethnographic study to determine how social workers function in the inner city it would be a logical development to plan techniques of data collection that involved both observation and interview techniques. She might add a review of records to this and state that overall she is using triangulation, looking at the same issues from multiple perspectives.

Alternatively, if Vivienne wished to focus more on what it feels like to be a social worker in the inner city, she might choose just to do interviews, because you cannot observe how people feel. If you say in the design section that you are going to undertake a phenomenological study, do not then go on to describe a process of data collection that is observational.

It is quite acceptable to state the intended location of the study in a research proposal because at this stage you won't be breaching any confidences if you do so. If, like Vivienne, you are going to complete the study in a stated local social services office, it is acceptable to say so – particularly if this is appropriate to the purpose of writing the proposal, for example, seeking funds from a local source. This may actually be necessary in order to indicate later who will be giving permission for you to complete the study.

Sometimes in qualitative research design, however, it is difficult to be very specific about the location. For example, if you choose to undertake an opportunistic sampling approach using a snowball technique (see Session Two) there may not be one single location for the study. You might be approaching people in several different locations which are yet to be decided.

It can also sometimes be difficult to be specific about the sample, for example, if there is no intention at the outset to specify an exact sample size, because the researcher is planning to determine how big the sample should be on the basis of saturation of categories. This is an area that requires careful consideration, particularly if submitting projects to an external committee more used to reading quantitative research with its associated larger numbers and related statistical tests.

The same consideration applies to data analysis. It is not uncommon for newcomers to research to get the idea that they need to mention statistics somewhere in a research proposal. They suddenly introduce these as the chosen form of analysis, even where they are totally inappropriate, for example where the data are in the form of words. Make sure, then, that the data analysis method chosen matches the method of data-collection being used. As we saw in Session Four, a study using semi-structured or open approaches to data collection will generate words – which will require some form of content analysis.

As we have noted throughout the text, there are more potential ethical dilemmas in qualitative research than in quantitative research because of the nature of the interaction between the researcher and the situation. For example, if you were planning to do an observation study you might observe bad practice or if you were interviewing people about some aspect of their lives that turned out to be quite an emotional area for them you could introduce problems into their lives by raising these issues. In the case of Carrigan's study, it is possible that in interviewing people who have attempted suicide the researcher might have generated distress. This is something that should be thought about at the outset. It is not uncommon for people writing proposals covering sensitive areas to describe how they will offer support if any distress is generated as a result of their research.

The issue of access must also be considered. In Resource 2, Carrigan noted that he sought permission from relevant consultant and nursing staff. This may be the norm in hospital-based research, but you will need to check any local arrangements for research that might have been introduced with new NHS managerial structures in recent years. For example, it might be considered necessary not only to have permission from professional groups but also from the manager of a unit in which the research is to be completed. The same principles would apply in social work or in any other care institution. The systems for seeking access to clients must be clarified and the appropriate authority identified before you begin the research. There would be little value in completing a research proposal and getting funding to carry out a project if permission to proceed was not forthcoming.

As mentioned earlier, the general principles necessary in writing research reports are very similar to those covered in reading research reports. However, in writing a research proposal you may also need to consider a couple of extra issues – the time scales and costs involved in completing the research.

Time scales

It is helpful to establish a time frame in which you will undertake your research study and sometimes this may actually be prescribed for you. For example, if you are required to do a project as part of a research methods course then you may have to complete this within the academic year. Again, if funds have been made available to support a project over one year only, then your timing is set. Developing a time plan helps focus your activities in a co-ordinated way and can be done very simply by stating the time for the projects and setting each stage alongside as illustrated in *Figure 17*.

Months 1-3	Establish project; begin literature search; plan research design
Month 4	Pilot techniques of data collection
Months 5-7	Main study – data collection
Months 8-9	Data analysis
Month 10-12	Write report
Month 12	Submit report

Figure 17: Broad time schedule for research project.

Project cost

Costing a project is complex and we can only touch on the subject here. If you are doing a funded project an accountant might well have some input into managing this. However, it is a useful exercise to carry out even if you are not seeking funds, because it serves to illustrate how costly research can be and prepares you for a time when you might need to do it in earnest.

The kind of factors you would need to consider are indicated in *Figure 18*.

	Cost in £
Researcher time	....
Secretarial support	....
Computer hire or purchase	....
Equipment – tape recorder	....
Travel to research site	....
Stationery and photocopying	....

Figure 18: Areas to consider when costing a research project.

You now have an opportunity to write a research proposal.

ACTIVITY 39   ALLOW **1** HOUR

Take a topic that interests you and, using the general principles for writing a research proposal outlined in *Table 11*, make a plan for a research proposal for a qualitative research study. Use no more than 1,000 words. This should give you enough space to allocate 100-200 words per section. Do not attempt to do a costing for this exercise.

Commentary

Since we cannot give you feedback on your specific proposal, you should make time to discuss what you have produced with a tutor, mentor or colleague with experience in this area.

Your proposal should address the following main issues:

- outcomes of the research project
- the nature of the proposed research
- background to the research
- methodology to be employed
- timescale
- design.

Summary

1 In this final session of the unit, we have considered how to write a research project proposal for qualitative design.

2 We began by considering the benefits of adopting a systematic approach towards planning a research proposal.

3 Before writing a proposal we considered the importance of ensuring clarity about the area of research.

4 The content of a research proposal was explored under generic headings.

Before you move on, check that you have achieved the objectives given at the beginning of this session and, if not, review the appropriate sections.

LEARNING REVIEW

You can use the list of learning outcomes given below to test the progress you have made in this unit. The list is an exact repeat of the one you completed in the beginning. You should tick the box on the scale that corresponds with the point you have reached now and then compare it with your scores on the learning profile you completed at the beginning of the study. If there are any areas you are still unsure about you might like to review the sessions concerned.

	Not at all	Partly	Quite well	Very well

Session One

I can:

	Not at all	Partly	Quite well	Very well
identify the influences which shape our views of the world	☐	☐	☐	☐
distinguish between inductive and deductive reasoning in research	☐	☐	☐	☐
explain how inductive and deductive reasoning influence theory development.	☐	☐	☐	☐

Session Two

I can:

	Not at all	Partly	Quite well	Very well
describe the basic principles of qualitative design	☐	☐	☐	☐
discuss a range of different approaches to qualitative research design	☐	☐	☐	☐
match research questions to an appropriate research design	☐	☐	☐	☐
explain what is meant by the term 'triangulation'	☐	☐	☐	☐
discuss the concepts of validity and reliability in the context of qualitative research	☐	☐	☐	☐
outline the potential ethical dilemmas researchers may face when completing qualitative research studies.	☐	☐	☐	☐

Session Three

I can:

	Not at all	Partly	Quite well	Very well
identify when it is appropriate to use interview techniques to collect data	☐	☐	☐	☐
explain the stages involved in collecting data via interviews	☐	☐	☐	☐

	Not at all	Partly	Quite well	Very well

Session three *continued*

- discuss the strengths and weaknesses of the interview approach ☐ ☐ ☐ ☐
- establish when it is appropriate to use observation techniques to collect data ☐ ☐ ☐ ☐
- outline how data can be collected through observation ☐ ☐ ☐ ☐
- describe the strengths and weaknesses of the observational approach. ☐ ☐ ☐ ☐

Session Four

I can:

- describe how data collected in qualitative studies can be broken down into data display, reduction and interpretation ☐ ☐ ☐ ☐
- explain how to undertake content analysis ☐ ☐ ☐ ☐
- report findings from qualitative research ☐ ☐ ☐ ☐
- recognise how to analyse data in different approaches to qualitative research. ☐ ☐ ☐ ☐

Session Five

I can:

- critically read a published research study that has used qualitative research design ☐ ☐ ☐ ☐
- distinguish between research reports that have a descriptive/exploratory orientation and those which have an interpretative orientation of ethnography, phenomenology and grounded theory ☐ ☐ ☐ ☐
- discuss how qualitative research can be used to influence practice and further development of knowledge. ☐ ☐ ☐ ☐

Session Six

I can:

- plan a research study using a qualitative approach ☐ ☐ ☐ ☐
- write a research proposal for qualitative design. ☐ ☐ ☐ ☐

Resources Section

Contents

Page

1 The strengths and weaknesses of quantitative and qualitative research: what method for nursing?   100

2 The psychosocial needs of patients who have attempted suicide by overdose   106

RESOURCE I

Journal of Advanced Nursing, (1994, 20, 716–721)

The strengths and weaknesses of quantitative and qualitative research: what method for nursing?

The overall purpose of research for any profession is to discover the truth of the discipline. This paper examines the controversy over the methods by which truth is obtained, by examining the differences and similarities between quantitative and qualitative research. The historically negative bias against qualitative research is discussed, as well as the strengths and weaknesses of both approaches, with issues highlighted by reference to nursing research. Consideration is given to issues of sampling; the relationship between the researcher and subject; methodologies and collated data; validity; reliability, and ethical dilemmas. The author identifies that neither approach is superior to the other; qualitative research papers are invaluable for the exploration of subjective experiences of patients and nurses, and quantitative methods facilitate the discovery of quantifiable information. Combining the strengths of both approaches in triangulation, if time and money permit, is also proposed as a valuable means of discovering the truth about nursing. It is argued that if nursing scholars limit themselves to one method of enquiry, restrictions will be placed on the development of nursing knowledge.

Defining quantitative and qualitative research

Quantitative research is also described by the terms 'empiricism' (Leach 1990) and 'positivism' (Duffy 1985). It derives from the scientific method used in the physical sciences (Cormack 1991). This research approach is an objective, formal, systematic process in which numerical data are used to quantify or measure phenomena and produce findings. It describes, tests and examines cause and effect relationships (Burns & Grove 1987), using a deductive process of knowledge attainment (Duffy 1985).

Whereas quantitative methodologies test theory deductively from existing knowledge, through developing hypothesized relationships and proposed outcomes for study, qualitative researchers are guided by certain ideas, perspectives or hunches regarding the subject to be investigated (Cormack 1991). Qualitative research also differs from quantitative approaches as it develops theory inductively. There is no explicit intention to count or quantify the findings, which are instead described in the language employed during the research process (Leach 1990). A qualitative approach is used as a vehicle for studying the empirical world from the perspective of the subject, not the researcher (Duffy 1987). Benoliel (1985), expands on this aspect and describes qualitative research as 'Modes of systematic enquiry concerned with understanding human beings and the nature of their transactions with themselves and with their surroundings'.

The aim of qualitative research is to describe certain aspects of a phenomenon, with a view to explaining the subject of study (Cormack 1991). The methodology itself is also described as phenomenology (Duffy 1985), or as a humanistic and idealistic approach (Leach 1990), with its origins lying in the disciplines of history, philosophy, anthropology, sociology and psychology (Cormack 1991). This historical foundation, which is not that of the physical science domain, has been cited as one of the great weaknesses of qualitative research, and is associated with the poor initial uptake of the approach within nursing (Bockmon & Rieman 1987).

Historical bias

Historically the use of true experiments has contributed greatly to the universal knowledge now acquired, especially in the field of medicine. The quantitative methods used produced legitimate scientific answers, and as a result of this 'hard' data, action was generated and changes took place (Melia 1982). The qualitative approaches produced 'soft' data which were, and are still described by some, as being inadequate in providing answers and generating any changes. One can argue that the use of the labels 'hard' and 'soft' data suggests in itself that analysis by numbers is of a superior quality to analysis by words (Corner 1991).

Benoliel (1985) considers the role nursing literature has played in giving qualitative research a lower status. The message, only 9 years ago, was that qualitative research was primarily for the discovery of knowledge to be tested, and was subsidiary to quantitative research. Bockmon & Rieman (1987) discussed the difficulties qualitative researchers had before the mid-1980s in achieving publication in traditional nursing journals. Historically, funding for research was awarded mainly to quantitative research reports (Duffy 1986), emphasizing the depth of acceptance and respect for this particular method.

Qualitative research thus has had a major obstacle to overcome in achieving recognition for its contribution to knowledge. Evaluation of qualitative research has been inhibited through lack of published papers. It is because of the recent increase in nursing publications using the qualitative methodology, that an analysis of the strengths and weaknesses of both quantitative and qualitative approaches can be conducted.

Sampling

Sampling procedures for each methodology are complex and must meet the criteria of the data collection strategy. Both research approaches require a sample to be identified which is representative of a larger population of people or objects. Quantitative research demands random selection of the sample from the study population and the random assignment of the sample to the various study groups (Duffy 1985). Statistical sampling relies on the study sample to develop general laws which can be generalized to the larger population. The advantage of results obtained from random sampling is that the findings have an increased likelihood of being generalizable. The disadvantage, and a weakness of the quantitative approach, is that random selection is time-consuming, with the result that many studies use more easily obtained opportunistic samples (Duffy 1985). This inhibits the possibilities of generalization, especially if the sample is too small. This is demonstrated in the study by Gould (1985) who investigated nurses' knowledge of isolation procedures within a specific health district. The study makes interesting comments, but it is not possible to generalize from its findings as the sample is too small.

Qualitative research, because of the in-depth nature of studies and the analysis of the data required, usually relates to a small, selective sample (Cormack 1991). A weakness of this can be the suspicion that the researcher could have been influenced by a particular predisposition, affecting the generalizability of the small scale study (Bryman 1988). This suggests that qualitative research has a low population validity. However, the strength of this approach is seen when the sample is well defined, for then it can be generalized to a population at large (Hinton

1987). Raggucci's (1972) ethnographic nursing study demonstrated the value of this approach in studying the benefits and practices of minority ethnic groups.

Relationship between researcher and subject

Relationship in quantitative research

In quantitative research the investigators maintain a detached, objective view in order to understand the facts (Duffy 1986). The use of some methods may require no direct contact with subjects at all, as in postal questionnaire surveys. It can be argued that even interview surveys require the researcher to have little, if any contact with respondents, especially if hired staff carry out most of the interviews (Bryman 1988). The strength of such a detached approach is avoidance of researcher involvement, guarding against biasing the study and ensuring objectivity.

Such an approach was successfully used in the West Berkshire-based perineal management trials of Sleep *et al*. (1984). This midwifery study was indirectly controlled by the researchers whose main involvement, other than randomly allocating mothers to either the controlled or experimental episiotomy group, was to analyse the data, once collected. The findings of this study, through its objectivity, have contributed to knowledge within this field.

Spencer (1983) argues that little is derived from such an indirect researcher-subject relationship especially in the health care setting. His major criticism is that the detached approach treats the participants as though they are objects and, as such, places hospitals on a par with car repair garages. Cormack (1991) also emphasizes the weaknesses of such an approach. She argues that the research participants are usually kept in the dark about the study, and are often left untouched by the research itself but are expected to transfer the findings into practice. These arguments are examples of the criticism that quantitative methods treat people merely as a source of data.

Researcher-subject relationship in qualitative research

As with quantitative research, qualitative methodologies also have supposed strengths and weaknesses regarding the closeness of the relationship between researcher and respondent. Duffy (1986) argues that a strength of such an interactive relationship is that the researcher obtains first-hand experience providing valuable meaningful data. As the researcher and the subject spend more time together the data are more likely to be honest and valid (Bryman 1988).

Supporting this argument is the study by Baruch (1981) which revealed that time and the subsequent relationship built between the researcher and the subjects was crucial for a genuine understanding of the dilemma faced by parents of sick or handicapped children. This appears to be a major strength of the qualitative approach itself, as Woodhouse & Livingwood (1991) pointed out in their study of a multi-agency substance abuse project. They claimed that the approach, because of the interactive method, far exceeded expected evaluation outcomes, by contributing to empowerment, and enhanced communication and clarification of roles among the partners involved in the project.

The weakness of such a close relationship is the likelihood that it may become pseudotherapeutic, complicating the research process and extending the responsibilities of the researcher (Ramos 1989). The possibility of becoming enmeshed with subjects could also lead to researchers having difficulty in separating their own experiences from those of their subjects (Sandelowski 1986) resulting in subjectivity (Cormack 1991). In its most extreme form this is referred to as 'going native', where the researcher loses awareness of being a researcher and becomes a participant (Bryman 1988). However this may not be entirely negative in that it facilitates a better understanding of the subject, as demonstrated by Oakley (1984).

Methodology

The research processes used in the quantitative approach include descriptive, correlational, quasi-experimental and experimental research (Cormack 1991). The strengths of such methods are that both true experiments and quasi-experiments provide sufficient information about the relationship between the variables under investigation to enable prediction and control over future outcomes. This is achieved by the ability of the researcher to manipulate an independent variable in order to study its effects on the dependent variable.

This strength can also be argued to be the weakness of the quantitative method, especially where nursing research is concerned. The methodology dismisses the experiences of the individual as unimportant, which is demonstrated in the Bockmon & Rieman study (1987), and regards human beings as merely reacting and responding to the environment (Cormack 1991). This causes difficulties in nursing research, because nursing uses an holistic view of people and their environment and, according to Broines & Cecchini (1991), quantitative methods do not permit this approach.

The qualitative approach includes methods such as grounded theory and ethnographic research (Denzin 1978). The strength of the methodology employed lies in the fact that it has an holistic focus, allowing for flexibility and the attainment of a deeper,

more valid understanding of the subject than could be achieved through a more rigid approach (Duffy 1986). It also allows subjects to raise issues and topics which the researcher might not have included in a structured research design, adding to the quality of data collected. The study by Melia (1982) is a good example of these strengths, and its findings have contributed to the knowledge of student nurses' perspectives on nursing.

A weakness of qualitative methodology is the possible effect of the researchers' presence on the people they are studying. As previously highlighted, the relationship between the researcher and participants may actually distort findings.

Data

The data collected in quantitative research are, as mentioned, hard and numerical. The strength of producing numbers as data is that this demonstrates an ordered system. Such an approach could be viewed as being necessary in an organization as big as the NHS, for as Spencer (1983) suggests, preparing an off-duty rota for 5000 employees needs quantitative methods and a computer. This argument is also supported by Kileen's (1984) study regarding new mothers where there was a need to use numerical data to identify the nursing resources needed, number of nurses involved, and what difference they made to patient outcome, length of stay, cost-effectiveness of discharge planning and the length of time the patients stayed out of hospital before any re-admission.

The opposing argument, suggesting the invalidity of numerical findings, is that data not displaying significance are often neglected, or alternatively attention is centred on a minority of the respondents leaving the majority unexplored; in other words there are 'deviant cases' (Cormack 1991). This therefore distorts the evaluation of data.

In contrast, the soft data collected in qualitative research identify and account for any 'deviant cases' (Cormack 1991). The rich data produced provide an illuminating picture of the subject, with great attention often given to pointing out intricate details. Evidence of this is seen in the study by Melia (1982) where student nurses' comments are quoted, enabling the reader to fully understand the subject being investigated.

The comparative weakness of qualitative data concerns the likelihood that some researchers can become overwhelmed by the data collected. They may become confused by their inability to limit the scope of the study, concentrating on a few manageable areas (Bryman 1988). In this situation the research can become poorly focused and ineffective.

Reliability

Quantitative research is considered more reliable than qualitative investigation. This is because a quantitative approach aims to control or eliminate extraneous variables within the internal structure of the study, and the data produced can also be assessed by standardized testing (Duffy 1985). This quantitative strength can be seen in the comparative analysis of patients' and nurses' perceptions about nursing activities in a postpartum unit, conducted by Morales-Mann (1989).

However, one can question the reliability of quantitative research, especially when the data have been stripped from the natural context, or there have been random or accidental events which are assumed not to have happened (Corner 1991).

The reliability of qualitative research is weakened by the fact that the process is under-standardized and relies on the insights and the abilities of the observer, thus making an assessment of reliability difficult (Duffy 1985). The study of Hind et al. (1990) examined this issue and demonstrated that reliability could be assessed by using independent experts to examine various aspects of the process of developing grounded theory. However, one must question the feasibility of employing such a costly process, both in terms of time and money, to verify the reliability of a qualitative study.

Validity

Although qualitative methodologies may have greater problems with reliability than quantitative methodologies, the position is reversed when the issue is validity. The weakness in quantitative research is that the more tightly controlled the study, the more difficult it becomes to confirm that the research situation is like real life. The very components of scientific research that demand control of variables can therefore be argued as operating against external validity and subsequent generalizability (Sandelowski 1986). Campbell & Stanley (1963) maintain that the more similar the research experiment is to the natural setting the greater is the validity and thus generalizability of the findings. The field studies concerning perineal management by Sleep et al. (1984) (also, Sleep 1984a,b) all contribute to the scientific understanding of this aspect of nursing. One reason that this can be claimed lies in the fact that the studies took place in a clinical environment, which increased validity.

The strength of qualitative research is proposed in the claim that there are fewer threats to external validity, because subjects are studied in their natural setting and encounter fewer controlling factors compared with quantitative research conditions (Sandelowski 1986). The researchers also become so immersed in the context and subjective states of the research subjects that they are able to give the assurance that the data are representative of the subject being studied, as seen in Oakley's (1984) antenatal clinic study. Paradoxically, the closeness of researchers also threatens the validity of the study if they become unable to maintain the distance required to describe or interpret experiences in a meaningful way, as discussed above (Hinton 1987). It is argued, however, that this is worth risking because of the high level of validity achieved by employing qualitative methodologies (Duffy 1985).

Ethical issues

Conceptually, the ethical considerations for both quantitative and qualitative research are the same: safety and protection of human rights. These are mainly achieved by using the process of informed consent. The utilization of informed consent is problematic in quantitative research, but practically impossible in qualitative methodologies in which the direction that the research takes is largely unknown (Ramos 1989). Munhall (1988) argues that informed consent can be achieved in qualitative research by re-negotiation when unexpected events occur, but one can argue in turn that this places greater responsibility on the researchers, as well as requiring them to possess a high level of skill, especially in negotiation.

The ethical weakness of quantitative research concerns the formulation of hypotheses. In nursing there are immense ethical considerations, especially for instance when it is explained that improvements will occur in patient care when a certain approach is adopted, and the eventual findings of the research do not support this. Dewis (1989) used a qualitative approach in her study of adolescents and young adults with spinal cord injuries, because of the absence of specific previous research and the ethical dilemma of formulating a hypothesis on assumptions. The qualitative approach, for this reason alone, proved valuable for this particular nursing study.

Discussion

For every strength there appears to be a corresponding weakness in both quantitative and qualitative research. It is this dilemma that has fuelled the debate over which approach is superior (Duffy 1986), and which method should therefore be adopted for nursing research. Nursing has a history of being divided; researchers in nursing can ill afford to be divided in attitudes to methodologies for this could add to the confusion and the division of the profession (Corner 1991). However, the author does not suggest that rigid uniformity about methodology should be the aim of nurse researchers, as studies have demonstrated that neither method has the upper hand or the complete set of answers.

Choosing just one methodology narrows a researcher's perspective, and deprives him or her of the benefits of building on the strengths inherent in a variety of research methodologies (Duffy 1986). Atwood (1985) disagreed with this, and argued that nursing should adopt quantitative approaches to build nursing into a science. He stated that this would provide nursing with a useful theory base with practical applications. Since this argument was posed by Atwood in 1985, studies have demonstrated that the model of measurement, prediction and causal inference does not easily fit a profession where health, illness adjustment, recovery, participation and care are frequently the variables to be measured whilst assessing the impact of nursing practice (Corner 1991). Relying solely on a quantitative approach to answer research questions has been seen to have serious limitations (Metcalfe 1983). Reliance solely on qualitative approaches has also been shown to have many limitations, although mainly of a different nature (Kileen 1984).

This debate could be seen as advantageous to nursing. Researchers are being forced to consider the controversial issues of both methodologies, and this requires them to have in-depth knowledge of epistemology and methodology and not to be restricted, as in the past, to the tradition of the physical sciences (Duffy 1985). Preference for a specific research strategy is not just a technical choice, it is an ethical, moral, ideological and political activity (Moccia 1988). This debate unearths these issues in relation to both approaches, allowing appropriate methods to be adopted by researchers in order to answer questions and develop nursing theories.

Considering the facts, it is argued that each approach should be evaluated in terms of its particular merits and limitations, in the light of the particular research question under study (Duffy 1987). However this implies that there are only technical differences between the two: those of research strategies and data collection procedures (Bryman 1988). There is a suggested alternative to this, that of combining the approaches, pulling on the strengths of each method and therefore countering the limitations posed by both. This research approach is called triangulation.

Triangulation

The main research areas that triangulation is concerned with are issues of data, investigator, theory and methodology (Murphy 1989). Morse (1991) argues that triangulation not only maximizes the strengths and minimizes the weaknesses of each approach,

but strengthens research results and contributes to theory and knowledge development. Silva & Rothbart (1984) hold a different opinion, arguing that a compromise resolution seems to ignore the significance of work presented that acknowledges various philosophies of science as factors in research and theory development. The literature demonstrates that there is no agreement between researchers about triangulation. This is not surprising when there is no agreement either about quantitative or qualitative methods employed within the approach.

The triangulation study conducted by Corner (1991) concerning newly registered nurses' attitudes to and educational preparation for caring for patients with cancer, illustrates both the strengths and weaknesses of the approach.

The study revealed a richer and deeper understanding of the subject matter than would otherwise be possible. Quantitative and qualitative approaches were found to complement each other while the inadequacies of each were actually offset. However, it also highlighted the time and cost implications: the volume of data produced was immense and an extremely broad knowledge base was required to analyse it, which meant that other researchers were contracted in to work on different parts of the analysis. These findings are similar to those of Murphy (1989) who used the method of triangulation to study traumatic life events.

Considering the evidence, it seems reasonable to suggest that triangulation is not the way forward for all nursing research but that it may help nursing to remove itself from the bipolar debate and restrictions, especially in the light of current financial constraints on health professions.

Conclusion

Although quantitative and qualitative methods are different, one approach is not superior to the other; both have recognized strengths and weaknesses and are used ideally in combination. It can therefore be argued that there is no one best method of developing knowledge, and that exclusively valuing one method restricts the ability to progress beyond its inherent boundaries. Recognizing the tension between researchers about quantitative and qualitative research, and attempting to understand it, may serve to create relevant and distinctive modes of enquiry in nursing. It may also help the unification rather than the division of nursing scholars.

From examining research in nursing, qualitative approaches appear to be invaluable for the exploration of subjective experiences of patients and nurses, while quantitative methods facilitate the development of quantifiable information. Combining the strengths of the methods in triangulation, if time and money permit results in the creation of even richer and deeper research findings. It seems that nursing research has the potential to provide a valuable resource for the health care system. As nursing discovers and uses different methodologies, it will assist in creating the necessary balance in the knowledge required to develop nursing as both a science and an art.

References

Atwood J.R. (1985) Advancing nursing science: quantitative approaches. *Western Journal of Nursing Research* **6**(3) Suppl., 9-15.

Baruch G. (1981) Moral tales: parents' stories of encounters with the health profession. *Sociology of Health and Illness* **3**(3), 275-296.

Benoliel J.Q. (1985) Advancing nursing science: qualitative approaches. *Western Journal of Nursing Research* **6**(3) Suppl., 1-8.

Bockmon D.F. & Rieman D.J. (1987) Qualitative versus quantitative nursing research. *Holistic Nursing Practice* **2**(1), 71-75.

Broines T.L. & Cecchini, D. (1991) Nursing versus medical research. *Heart and Lung* **20**(2), 206-207.

Bryman A. (1988) *Quantity and Quality in Social Research*. Routledge, London.

Burns N. & Grove S.K. (1987) *The Practice of Nursing Research: Conduct, Critique and Utilization*. W.B. Saunders, Philadelphia.

Campbell D.T. & Stanley J.C. (1963) *Experimental and quasi-experimental design for research*. Rand McNally, Chicago.

Clark E. (1988) *Research Awareness 9: The Experimental Perspective*. Ashford, Southampton.

Cormack D.F.S. (ed.) (1991) *The Research Process in Nursing* 2nd edn. Blackwell Scientific, Oxford.

Corner J. (1991) In search of more complete answers to research questions. Quantitative versus qualitative research methods: is there a way forward? *Journal of Advanced Nursing* **16**(3), 718-727.

Denzin N.K. (1978) *The Research Act: A Theoretical Introduction to Sociological Methods*. McGraw-Hill, London.

Dewis M.E. (1989) Spinal cord injured adolescents and young adults: the meaning of body changes. *Journal of Advanced Nursing* **4**(5), 389-396.

Duffy M.E. (1985) Designing nursing research: the qualitative-quantitative debate. *Journal of Advanced Nursing* **10**(3), 225-232.

Duffy M.E. (1986) Quantitative and qualitative research: antagonistic or complementary? *Nursing and Health Care* **8**(6), 356-357.

Duffy M.E. (1987) Methodological triangulation: a vehicle for merging quantitative and qualitative methods. *Image* **19**(3), 130-133.

Gould D. (1985) Isolation procedures in one health district. *Nursing Times* **81**(7), 47-50.

Hind P.S., Scandrett-Hibden & McCaulay L.S. (1990) Further assessment of method to estimate reliability and validity of qualitative research findings. *Journal of Advanced Nursing* **15**(4), 430-435.

Hinton A. (1987) *Research Awareness 7: the Ethnographic Perspective*. Ashford, Southampton.

Kileen M. (1984) From hospitals to home: continuous care for new mothers and infants. *Nursing Management* **15**(3), 10-13.

Leach M. (1990) Philosophical choice. Nursing: *The Journal of Clinical Practice, Education and Management* **4**(3), 16-18.

Melia K.M. (1982) 'Tell it as it is' – qualitative methodology and nursing research: understanding the student nurse's world. *Journal of Advanced Nursing* **7**(4), 327-335.

Metcalfe C. (1983) A study of change in the method of organising the delivery of nursing care in a ward of a maternity hospital. In *Nursing Research: Studies in Patient Care* (Wilson-Barnet J. ed.), John Wiley, Chichester, pp. 119-140.

Moccia P. (1988) A critique of compromise: beyond the methods debate. *Advanced Nursing Science* **10**(4), 1-9.

Morales-Mann E.T. (1989) Comparative analysis of the perceptions of patients and nurses about the importance of nursing activities in a postpartum unit. *Journal of Advanced Nursing* **14**(6), 478-484.

Morse J.M. (1991) Approaches to qualitative and quantitative methodological triangulation. *Nursing Research* **40**(1), 120-123.

Munhall P.L. (1988) Ethical considerations in qualitative research. *Western Journal of Nursing Research* **10**(2), 150-162.

Murphy S.A. (1989) Multiple triangulation. Application in a programme of nursing research. *Nursing Research* **38**(5), 291-297.

Oakley A. (1984) *Taking It Like A Woman*. Cape, London.

Raggucci A.T. (1972) The ethnographic approach and nursing research. *Nursing Research* **21**(6), 485-490.

Ramos M.C. (1989) Some ethical implications of qualitative research. *Research in Nursing and Health* **12**(1), 57-63.

Sandelowski M. (1986) The problem of rigor in qualitative research. *Advances in Nursing Science* **8**(3), 27-37.

Silva M.C. & Rothbart D. (1984) An analysis of changing trends in philosophies of science on nursing theory development and testing. *Advanced Nursing Science* **6**(2), 1-13.

Sleep J., Grant J., Elbourne D., Spencer J. &

Chalmers I. (1984) West Berkshire perineal management trial. *British Medical Journal* 289(6445), 587-590.

Sleep J. (1984a) Episiotomy in normal delivery. *Nursing Times* 80(47), 28-30.

Sleep J. (1984b) Management of the perineum. *Nursing Times* 80(48), 51-54.

Spencer J. (1983) Research with the human touch. *Nursing Times* 29(12), 24-27.

Woodhouse L.D. & Livingwood W.C. (1991) Exploring the versatility of qualitative design for evaluating community substance abuse protection projects. *Qualitative Health Research* 1(4), 434-445.

RESOURCE 2

Journal of Advanced Nursing ,(1994, 20, 635-642)

The psychosocial needs of patients who have attempted suicide by overdose

This is an exploratory study using qualitative methods to investigate and highlight psychosocial needs as perceived by individuals who have survived an attempted suicide through self-poisoning. Respondents consisted of a convenience sample of six people (three male and three female). Data were collected through interviews and analysed using the principles of content analysis devised by Field and Morse. Major needs identified include the need to have control of one's life and the need to be supported. Findings indicate that these needs are not being met by the current mental health care delivery system. In addition, nurses must begin to pay greater attention to assessment and planning of care for this group of patients. A wider use of psychosocial therapies such as crisis intervention and family therapy are urgently required. Above all there is a need for more in-depth understanding and improved communication with patients who have attempted suicide by self-poisoning.

Introduction

In the past decade there has been a steady increase in the number of deaths from suicide in Northern Ireland. Since 1980 the number has increased from 5.2 per 100,000 of the population to 9.9 per 100,000 of the population in 1990 (DHSS 1981-1991). Not only does the problem of suicide pose a major challenge for our health care services but so does the increased incidence of deliberate self-harm. Since the 1960s the number of people presenting in accident and emergency departments with deliberate self-harm has steadily increased (Hawton 1983, Hawton & Catalan 1987, Coleman 1989).

The most common method used in deliberate self-harm is that of poisoning. Every year over 100,000 people take an overdose of tablets in the United Kingdom (Hawton & Catalan 1987, Coleman 1989, Gelder *et al.* 1989). In one hospital alone in Northern Ireland there were 282 overdose admissions from December 1990 to September 1991 (unpublished report, Resource Management Support Office, Londonderry). A more frightening aspect perhaps is that this phenomenon is more common among young adults (Newnes 1982, Coleman 1989).

A diagnosis of overdose of tablets is now the most frequent single reason for admission of women to medical wards, and among men it is second only to that of chronic heart disease (Hawton & Catalan 1987, Gelder *et al.* 1989, Coleman 1989).

Dunleavey (1992) suggests that in the past it was all too easy to dismiss parasuicide patients as 'psychiatric cases'. Gorman & Masterton (1990) support this by suggesting that the problem of attempted suicide is complex and diverse and is more strongly associated with social factors than mental illness *per se*. Hawton & Catalan (1987) suggest that prevention of further episodes of self-poisoning continues to be a problem. Repeated readmission to hospital can easily become the norm for these patients.

Prevention

In 1984 the Department of Health and Social Services (DHSS) in Northern Ireland issued a document entitled *The Management of Deliberate Self-Harm*. This document stated that much more needs to be known about the prevention of self-poisoning. It was also recognized that more research was needed to establish the most effective patterns of care for patients who have deliberately harmed themselves. Various recommendations were put forward by the working groups including:

1   the evaluation of the psychiatric and social state of every patient admitted

with this diagnosis;

2 a psychosocial assessment to be carried out on patients by staff specifically trained for this task; and

3 after care of patients by community psychiatric nurses or other specially trained nurses in collaboration with the general practitioner.

Evidence to date, however, does not suggest that these recommendations have had any impact upon repetition rates (Hawton & Catalan 1987). In addition there is also a need for further work to build upon the findings of Dunleavey (1992) who suggests that patients admitted to hospital following attempted suicide present a real challenge to nurses.

Theoretical perspectives

Developmental theories – psychoanalytic

Freud (1957), in his attempt to explain suicidal acts, believed that irrational behaviour resulted largely from internal conflicts between sexual or aggressive impulses and the demands of one's conscience and reality. These internal conflicts resulted in a turning of aggressive impulses against the self with self-destructive behaviour being the end result.

Application of this perspective to nursing practice would entail the nurse conducting a series of interviews to explore and bring to the fore these conflicts. This would involve reconstruction of early childhood experiences in an attempt to unearth and deal with the sources of conflict. However, the psychoanalytic model has been criticized for its limited treatment role in the sense that its theory is based, to a large extent, on early childhood experiences and is often considered to be somewhat outdated (Wilson & Kneisel 1988, Stuart & Sundine 1991).

Nevertheless, Robinson (1983) argues that the nurse can better understand the philosophy underpinning psychiatric nursing through the psychodynamic perspective. Although reference is made to this approach to care within the nursing curriculum, few nurses would have undergone specialized training (Fabricius 1991). It is, therefore, important for nurses to learn the language of and ideas about psychodynamics in order to be valued as theorists and participate as equal members of the psychiatric team (Wilson & Kneisel 1988).

Psychosocial perspective

Leonard (1967) has made strong reference to Erikson when she proposed a developmental theory of suicide and attempted suicide. She suggested that the second and third years of life are crucial for the development of suicidal tendencies. Leonard (1967) asserts that it is during these years that a child begins his/her struggle for independence and autonomy from the mother. During these years conflict can arise when the child is torn between dependence on the mother and independence from the mother. She suggests that this conflict can be resolved in different ways, each of which is associated with a kind of suicidal tendency.

Although Leonard's (1967) theory on suicide does offer some stimulating ideas to nursing, it is, nevertheless, limited in the sense that it is totally developmental in nature. Unlike Erikson (1987) she places a lot of emphasis on the first three years of life but fails to give much consideration to other ages and stages of development. Erikson on the other hand, whilst psychoanalytical in his approach, places greater emphasis on the social perspective of development throughout the life span.

Fitzpatrick *et al.* (1982) suggest that in applying Erikson's approach to the suicidal individual the nurse would focus on the level of organization and interaction of the id, ego and superego and the level of development.

The goal of nursing intervention would be to help the individual resolve the conflict and continue to develop through the psychosocial stages as outlined by Erikson (1987).

Stressful life events theory

Many researchers have in the past based their studies on the stressful life events theory and they have produced evidence to suggest that suicide or attempted suicide follows if the individual has a reduced ability to cope with the major life events (Holmes & Rahe 1967, Morgan 1979, Farmer & Creed 1989). However, in a study by Lazarus (1981) 'little hassles' were found to have an impact on health also. Lazarus (1981) suggests that these little hassles can range from getting stuck in a traffic jam to an argument with a teenage son. He suggests that daily hassles are more closely linked to and may have a greater effect on our moods and our health than the major misfortunes of life.

Stressful life events, if not successfully managed, can bring about a crisis in one's life. Wilson & Kneisel (1988) suggest that a crisis is a situation in which customary problem solving or decision making methods are not adequate. Working with a helping person increases the likelihood that a crisis will be resolved in a positive way.

Fitzpatrick *et al.* (1982) suggest that King's (1971) model of nursing intervention is especially congruent with crisis intervention methodology. The model focuses on altering the individual's perception and cognition of the experience and the interaction with internal and external environments. In the case of an individual experiencing a crisis resulting from a stressful life event the nurse would assist the individual to take a fresh look at his/her perception and understanding of the situation. The nurse and patient would become engaged in mutual goal setting to resolve the crisis and develop new coping skills.

Stuart & Sundine (1991) assert that conclusions regarding life events theory are far from definite. They are critical of the theoretical and methodological aspects of research in this area with particular emphasis on validity and reliability of data collection methods. Another criticism levelled at this work is that the subjective evaluation of the significance of life events to the individual has often been neglected.

Social integration theory

Emile Durkheim (1975) attempted to explain suicidal behaviour from a sociological perspective. In order to do this he had to define the suicidal act as a social incident that would require explanation from a sociological stand point. Durkheim argued that by comparing the incidence of suicidal acts in different countries and among social groups within each country he could demonstrate the suicide rates were relatively constant. He concluded, therefore, that a collective tendency towards suicide existed (Thompson 1982).

Mullis & Byers (1987) cited two studies by Harris (1966) and Kumler (1964) to demonstrate the fact that nursing has for many years recognized the role of social support for suicide attempters. Indeed Wilson & Kneisel (1988) suggest that because nursing has been concerned with the social environment of the client for decades, the term social support might be seen as pouring old wine into new bottles. Nevertheless other writers on the subject have recognized the need to redefine the concept of social support and call for a more in-depth investigation focusing on its relevance to suicide prevention (Tolsdorf 1976, Norbeck 1982).

Each and every one of us is exposed to stressful situations of some degree on a daily basis (Lazarus 1981) and as a result we call on our social networks for support from time to time. Greenblath et al. (1982) suggest that social networks can act as social support systems to promote mental health and buffer psychological stress. In a similar study by Tolsdorf (1976) it was concluded that fundamental differences existed in not only the size of the network, but also the relationships that existed within the social network groups. The study reports psychiatric patients as perceiving their networks as cold and rejecting, unsympathetic, domineering or controlling. They also tended to have a history of not calling on their network for advice or support during periods of crisis.

In a more recent study by Hart et al. (1988) on suicidal behaviour and social networks, it was concluded that the size of the social networks of suicidal individuals are impaired relative to non-suicidal individuals. They go on to suggest that the interaction within the social networks was more effective for patients who had attempted suicide, but had no diagnosed psychiatric illness.

Speck (1967) suggests that the social network approach to therapy includes the friends, neighbours, relatives and fellow workers with whom the person in crisis has a social relationship. In the case of the suicidal individual the nurse can facilitate such interactions within the individual's own environment. Speck defines this as social network therapy and presents it as an extension to group therapy.

The study

The aim of the study was to investigate and highlight psychosocial needs, as perceived by individuals who have survived an attempt of deliberate self-poisoning. It also sets out to evaluate health care support received during and following the incident.

An exploratory, descriptive design was considered the most appropriate. Even though the collection of data may not go beyond describing the individual's perspective, there was the possibility that new findings might emerge and these could act as a basis for further study.

Focused interviews

Focused interviews proposed by Cohen and Manion (1989) were considered to be most appropriate since the respondents would be telling their story face to face with the interviewer and clarification of specific areas could be sought if need be. Even though some questions had been prepared in advance the interviews were non-directive to a point in that the order and content of questions were dependent on the individual's response. However, should the respondent wander off the subject, the interviewer would refocus them by asking a specific question which was previously prepared. A convenience sample of six respondents (three males and three females) was used.

Permission to conduct the interviews was sought and was subsequently granted by the Research Ethical Committee and appropriate health board. Permission was also sought and granted by the relevant physicians and charge nurses to interview patients who were admitted for treatment of drug overdose. Verbal permission to interview each respondent was obtained from them while they were in hospital for treatment following a drug overdose. At this stage it was also explained to each respondent how the researcher had obtained their names. A preliminary visit following discharge from hospital was requested at this stage so that a more detailed outline of the study could be given and any queries could be answered.

It was also felt that the respondents would be in a more stable position at this stage to accept or reject involvement in the study. A further interview was arranged with each respondent during the preliminary visit. All respondents were informed of the right to withdraw from the study at any time.

Data analysis

Data analysis was based on the principles of content analysis proposed by Field & Morse (1991). By using a combination of both 'manifest' and 'latent' content analysis it was possible to analyse data in the form of overall descriptions of messages and also to present the results in a descriptive fashion in order to outline the number of times specific concepts were observed – for example, four respondents expressed feelings of poor self-esteem.

Themes were identified and presented under the three main categories presented in the literature review, i.e. developmental theories, stressful life events and social integration.

Findings and discussion

All six respondents identified life events that have been described as major as classified by Farmer & Creed (1989). They included relationship problems and family problems. Four respondents made a direct association between the stressful life events identified by them and their attempted suicide.

1   'It's because of the problems that I am having that made me do this.'
2   'If my daddy stopped drinking I would stop feeling like this.'
3   'I split up with my wife and that was the last straw.'
4   'When you lose your job you lose everything.'

It is unclear, however, whether the life event itself or the cognitive appraisal of the event by the respondents had the greatest influence on their actions.

In the case of three respondents in particular, life events were associated with other problems such as loss of self-image, loss of control of life and communication needs. This would seem to indicate that these particular respondents perceived stress as a threat rather than a challenge and as a result were unable to cope effectively.

One respondent identified life events that, according to Lazarus (1981) could be described as minor or 'little hassles'. Reference was made to incidents such as a son smoking, a husband refusing to help with housework, and trying to help children with homework.

Lazarus (1981) argues that 'daily hassles' such as these are more closely linked to and

may have a greater effect on our moods and our health than the major misfortunes of life. Definite conclusions cannot be drawn as this was evident only in one case.

Overall, however, there is a clear need for nurses to be competent in identifying stressful life events in order to plan and implement the most appropriate methods of care aimed at reducing suicide attempts. Aguilera & Messick (1986) argue that crisis intervention, as a method, can offer the immediate help that a patient requires during a crisis in order to re-establish equilibrium.

Maintenance of self-esteem

Four respondents expressed feelings of poor self-esteem. One 19-year-old female made references to feelings of poor self-esteem as something that had been with her since childhood.

When I was at school I was a wee fat girl and I still am...everybody laughed at me because of my weight.

Erikson (1987) has argued that it is during the second and third years of life that a child has to cope with the crisis of autonomy versus shame and doubt. If the crisis is resolved in a constructive way the child learns to have self-control without loss of self-esteem. However, if the crisis is not resolved shame and doubt may result. He also asserts that significant others help to resolve developmental crises by satisfying the person's interpersonal needs and by conveying their interpretations of the meaning of the crisis.

Two respondents made reference to developmental problems in their lives, one to the poor relationship between her parents and the other to the fact that her mother was a domineering woman who made the decisions. These factors may have had some bearing on the personality development of the respondents.

Peplau (1988) suggests that children can be most unclear about their perceptions of self and have many feelings of inadequacy because of mother-father-child relationships.

Implications

From a nursing perspective it is indeed evident that patients with low self-esteem need professional support. Aguilera & Messick (1986) assert that when self-esteem is low, or when a situation is perceived as particularly threatening, the person is strongly in need of and seeks out others. The nurse, as the primary carer, should be in the ideal position to provide positive support and enhance self-esteem. In order to be able to foster this the nurse must be, in the first instance, competent in identifying and analysing feelings and as a result provide therapeutic nursing care in whatever form is most appropriate.

Stuart & Sundine (1991) assert that there

is a need for the nurse to delve beyond the objective and observable behaviours to the subjective and internal world of the patient. Only when the nurse explores this realm will the patient's actions be given meaning and negative actions such as suicide be prevented.

Need to be loved and have control of life

Five respondents expressed a need to be loved and wanted. This need seemed to be associated with the loss of self-esteem, powerlessness and with the development of stressful life events. Wilson & Kneisel (1988) suggest that individuals with low self-esteem are preoccupied with a sense of personal failure, guilt, hopelessness, pessimism, and unfavourable comparisons with others. This scenario was reflected in the interviews through phrases such as 'nobody cares about me, nobody seems to want me'. Lack of control of life was also reflected in phrases such as 'everything is my fault and how will I cope?' These findings seem to support Seligman's learned helplessness model (Seligman 1975) in the sense that there is no hope for the future and a belief that the patient cannot do anything to improve the situation.

The need to escape

All six respondents made reference to trying to get away from a crisis situation. However, this escape may not necessarily have been intended to result in death since only two of the six respondents made a direct reference to death. Hatton *et al.* (1977) suggest that attempted suicides do not always have death as their primary objective. These attempts are often viewed as a means of communicating and a cry for help (Beck *et al.* 1974, Dale 1980, Newnes 1982, Dunleavey 1992). This assertion has been supported to some extent since two respondents did make a reference to their attempt being 'a cry for help'. One man in his twenties stated, 'I was frightened when I had taken the tablets...I suppose deep down I didn't want to die.'

Although two respondents did not make reference to their attempt being a cry for help they, nevertheless, did not indicate that their intention was to die. This causes some confusion as to what their real intentions were. It must be emphasized that patients are often reluctant to indicate that their intention is to die (Hawton & Catalan 1987). Parasuicide is not exclusively about dying but also about survival and contact, its significance lies in the message it is intended to convey (Strengel 1977, Gibbs 1990, Dunleavey 1992).

Communication with professionals

Problems were highlighted by all six respondents regarding communication difficulties with either general practitioners, hospital doctors or nursing staff. The need for someone to listen to them and attempt to understand their feelings seemed to be of major importance. Although three respondents stated that nurses tried to understand them, reference was made on two occasions to the need for nurses to get involved at a deeper level. One girl in her teens stated, 'There was plenty I could have told them if they went about it a different way.' One could assume, therefore, that although nurses did seem to attempt to understand these patients' needs, their methods and approach (at least on two occasions) seemed to be unsatisfactory from the patient's perspective.

Skills such as listening were referred to by two respondents and the need for nurses to spend time with patients on three occasions. These findings are supported by Dunleavey's (1992) findings in a similar study when she reports that interactions with nursing staff were rare and were generally restricted to either physical care or superficial social chats, often amounting to little more than 'passing comments'. This points to the importance of more in-depth assessment of patients' psychosocial needs and to further development of nurses' interpersonal skills.

On one occasion reference was made to the nurse telling a patient that he would be alright and talking about general things to keep his mind occupied. This approach by nurses could be interpreted as being more related to custodial care than supportive care since the subject did refer to the fact that the nurse may have been 'making sure I wasn't thinking of doing it again'. By using this approach there may be a tendency for the nurse to interact less frequently and at a superficial level with the patient. This assertion is supported by Gibbs (1990) who suggests that professionals often express negative opinions about talking to patients who have attempted suicide, suggesting that if you talk too much they might do it again.

Five respondents stated that there was a need for better understanding and more assistance by nurses regarding individual difficulties with problem solving. One woman stated, 'Maybe they could see [the nurses] if I'm going wrong or who's going wrong in the house.' Aguilera & Messick (1986) suggest that the goal of crisis intervention is to help the individual gain an intellectual understanding of the relationship between crisis and the inability to communicate feelings. Through a combination of crisis intervention principles and nursing intervention the nurse could seek to assist the patient to communicate his/her feelings more effectively. This objective could be further enhanced through the careful choice of a nursing model. Fitzpatrick *et al.* (1982) argue that King's model of nursing intervention is especially congruent with crisis intervention methodology.

Professional assistance

Five respondents expressed the need for professional assistance/support following discharge from hospital. Although professional assistance was provided in four cases in this particular study, some dissatisfaction seemed to be present in relation to the quality of this assistance. Those respondents who expressed the need for more professional assistance also expressed a need for assistance with problem solving and communication. In a study by Bancroft *et al.* (1977) similar findings were reported. Although a high degree of contact with helping agencies was reported there seemed to be a need for more detailed investigation and analysis of types of relationships and communication problems.

Dunleavey (1992) reports evidence of infrequent and superficial communication between nurses and hospital in-patients who have attempted suicide. From the evidence available, therefore, there seems to be a need to further explore the quality of communication that exists between nurses and patients, both from a hospital ward and community perspective.

Relationship with family

Relationships with family members feature strongly throughout the interviews. These relationships were related to communication difficulties with close family members such as husband, wife, mother or father. Most difficulty seemed to relate to the inability to express emotions and get feedback from close family members. One respondent stated, 'I could never have talked to my father or mother about a broken relationship...they would have laughed at me.' Varadaraj *et al.* (1986) suggest that self-destructive acts could be considered as part and parcel of the dysfunctional communication systems that can exist between the patient and significant others. If a family communication problem is identified then the nurse could strive to improve the situation through a family therapy approach.

Stuart & Sundine (1991) suggest that the treatment goal of family therapy using communication theory is to correct pathological patterns of communication between family members in which members express themselves clearly and directly and ask for and receive feedback. However, Barker (1986) suggests that caution is required in some cases with family therapy since an alteration in the family situation could increase the stress faced by one or more individuals, and this could lead to a worsening of their condition with perhaps depression or even suicide resulting.

Social network therapy

There is a need for better support from the immediate family and the wider social perspective. This need seemed to be also related to stressful events in the patients' lives, low self-esteem and the need for better social integration. One can conclude, therefore, that if there is a causal relationship between these factors, social network therapy may have benefits. Wilson & Kneisel (1988) suggest that the goal of social network therapy is to bring together as many of the individual's social network contacts as possible in an attempt to support the individual through the crisis period. This in turn would possibly help to instil a positive feeling in the individual.

Vidalis *et al.* (1987) report a very high incidence (84%) of failure of self-poisoning patients to consistently attend out-patient treatment units. Although five of the six respondents in this particular study had out-patient appointments it is impossible at this stage to predict whether appointments would be consistently adhered to or not. Individuals may need that little bit of encouragement from helping agencies such as community nurses to continue to attend out-patient clinics. Dunleavey (1992) suggests that the smallest interventions can be of real benefit to these vulnerable people and the nurse's approach may play a pivotal role in patients' uptake of counselling or psychiatric support.

Limitations of the study

The small sample size used in the study is not representative of the total population of Northern Ireland. In some instances questions were rephrased during the interviews which could have influenced the nature of responses. Although every attempt was made to be as objective as possible some subjectivity may have influenced the development of categories during content analysis.

The length of time between discharge from hospital and the interviews varied between subjects from five days to six weeks. As a result the accuracy of information obtained in the interviews may have been reduced since a clear recollection of feelings and events may fade over time.

Some subjects refused to be interviewed or refused to stay in hospital. These subjects may have perceived themselves as having different or fewer needs than those who were interviewed. Despite these limitations, the study does provide valuable information on the psychosocial needs of a group of patients who have survived an attempted suicide through self-poisoning.

Conclusion

It is evident from these findings that the presence and/or cognitive appraisal of stressful life events by the respondents seems to have an influence on their actions. Many other needs seem to stem from the fact that the respondents are experiencing or have experienced a crisis or crises in their lives. From a nursing perspective there seems to be a need for more in-depth assessment of needs and more involvement of patients in planning their own care. A more widespread use of therapies that are geared towards assisting the patients to cope with and come to terms with their problems is required.

These therapies require a knowledge and application of developmental theories, stressful life events theory and social integration theory. Communication difficulties exist both from the nurses' and patients' perspectives and seem to be one of the key factors associated with improvement of patient care. In addition it has become evident from this research that people who have attempted suicide by self-poisoning should be involved in the review and recommendations of psychiatric services in the light of this escalating problem.

References

Aguilera D.C. & Messick J.M.L. (1986) *Crisis Intervention* 5th edn. C.V. Mosby, Toronto.

Bancroft J., Skrimshire A., Casson J., Harvard-Watts O. & Reynolds F. (1977) People who deliberately poison or injure themselves: their problems and their contacts with helping agencies. *Psychological Medicine* 7, 289-3-3.

Barker P. (1986) *Basic Family Therapy* 2nd edn. Collins Books, Oxford.

Beck A.T., Harvey L.D. & Dan J. (1974) *The Prediction of Suicide*. Charles Press, London.

Cohen L. & Manion L. (1989) *Research Methods in Education* 3rd edn. Croom Helm, Beckenham, Kent.

Coleman V. (1989) *The Health Scandal: Your Health in Crisis*. Mandarin Paperbacks, London.

Dale D. (1980) Suicide. Do the Samaritans really help? *Nursing Times* 75(45), 1981-1982.

Department of Health and Social Security (1981-1991) *Register General Northern Ireland Annual Reports*. Her Majesty's Stationery Office, Belfast.

Department of Health and Social Security (1984) *The Management of Deliberate Self-Harm*. Health Service Management, Her Majesty's Stationery Office, London.

Dunleavey R. (1992) An adequate response to a cry for help. Parasuicide patients' perceptions of their nursing care. *Professional Nurse* 7(4), 213-215.

Durkheim E. (1975) *Suicide: A Study in Sociology* (Translated by Spalding J.A. & Simpson G.: Simpson G. ed.) Routledge & Kegan Paul, London, pp. 297-392.

Erikson E. (1987) *Childhood and Society*. Paladin Grafton Books, London.

Fabricius J. (1991) Running on the spot or can nursing really change? *Psychoanalytic Psychotherapy* 5(2), 97-108.

Farmer R. & Creed F. (1989) Life events and hostility in self-poisoning. *British Journal of Psychiatry* 154, 390-395.

Field P.A. & Morse J.M. (1991) Nursing Research: *The Application of Qualitative Approaches*. Croom Helm, Beckenham, Kent.

Fitzpatrick J., Whall A., Johnston R. & Floyd J. (1982) *Nursing Models and their Psychiatric Mental Health Applications*. Prentice Hall, London.

Freud S. (1957) Mourning and melancholia. In the standard edition of *The Complete Psychological Works of Sigmond Freud*. Hogarth Press, London. Cited in Ullmann L.P. & Krashner L. (1975) *A Psychological Approach to Abnormal Behaviour*. Prentice Hall, Englewood Cliffs, New Jersey.

Gelder M., Gath D. & Mayou R. (1989) *Oxford Textbook of Psychiatry*. Oxford University Press, Oxford.

Gibbs A. (1990) Aspects of communication with people who have attempted suicide. *Journal of Advanced Nursing* 15, 1245-1249.

Gorman D. & Masterton G. (1990) General practice consultation patterns before and after intentional overdose: a matched control study. *British Journal of General Practice* 40(332), 102-105.

Greenblath M., Becerra R. & Serafetinides M.D. (1982) Social networks and mental health: an overview. *The American Journal of Psychiatry* 139(8), 977-984.

Harris R.A. (1966) Factors related to continued suicidal behaviour in dyadic relationships. *Nursing Research* 15, 72-75. Cited in Mullis M.R. & Byers P.H. (1987) Social support in suicidal inpatients. *Journal of Psychosocial Nursing* 25(4), 16-19.

Hart E.E., Williams C.L. & Davidson J.A. (1988) Suicidal behaviour, social networks and psychiatric diagnosis. *Social Psychiatry And Psychiatric Epidemiology* 23(4), 222-227.

Hatton C.L., Valente McBride S. & Rink A. (1977) *Suicide Assessment and Intervention*. Appleton Century Crofts, London.

Hawton K.E. (1983) Attempted suicide. *Medicine International* 1(33), 1551-1553.

Hawton K. & Catalan J. (1987) *Attempted Suicide. A Practical Guide to its Nature and Management*. Oxford University Press, Oxford.

Holmes T.H. & Rahe R. (1967) The social readjustment rating scale. *Journal of Psychosomatic Research* 11, 213-218.

King I.M. (1971) *Towards a Theory of Nursing*. Wiley & Sons, New York. Cited in Fitzpatrick J., Whall A., Johnston J. & Floyd J. (1982) *Nursing Models and their Psychiatric Mental Health Applications*. Prentice Hall, London.

Kumler F. (1964) Communications between

suicide attempters and significant others: an exploratory study. *Nursing Research* 13, 268-270. Cited in Mullis M.R. & Byers P.H. (1987) Social support in suicidal inpatients. *Journal Of Psychosocial Nursing* 25(4), 16-19.

Lazarus R.S. (1981) Little hazards can be hazardous to health. *Psychology Today* 15, 58-62.

Leonard C.V. (1967) *Understanding and Preventing Suicide*. Charles C. Thomas, Springfield, Illinois.

Morgan H.G. (1979) Death Wishes, *Understanding Management of Self-Harm*. Wiley, Chichester.

Mullis M.R. & Byers P.H. (1987) Social support in suicidal inpatients. *Journal of Psychosocial Nursing* 25(4), 16-19.

Newnes C. (1982) A cry for help. *Nursing Mirror* 154(6), 16-18.

Norbeck J.S. (1982) The use of social support in clinical practice. *Journal Of Psychosocial Nursing* 20, 22-29.

Peplau H.E. (1988) *Interpersonal Relations in Nursing*. Macmillan Education, London.

Robinson L. (1983) *Psychiatric Nursing as a Human Experience* 3rd edn. W.B. Saunders, London.

Seligman M.E.P. (1975) *Helplessness: On Depression, Development and Death*. W.H. Freeman, San Francisco.

Speck R.V. (1967) Psychotherapy of the social network of a schizophrenic family. *Family Processes* 6, 208-214.

Strengel E. (1977) *Suicide and Attempted Suicide*. Penguin Books, Harmondsworth.

Stuart C.W. & Sundine S.J. (1991) *Principles and Practice of Psychiatric Nursing*. C.V. Mosby, Toronto.

Thompson K. (1982) *Emile Durkheim*. Routledge, London.

Tolsdorf C.C. (1976) Social networks, support and coping. An exploratory study. *Family Processes* 15, 407-417.

Varadaraj R., Mendonca J.D. & Rauchenberg P.M. (1986) Motives and intent: a comparison of views of overdose patients and their key relatives/friends. *Canadian Journal of Psychiatry* 31(7), 621-624.

Vidalis A.A., Jungalwalla H.N. & Baker G.H.B. (1987) Self-poisoning: could psychiatric management be improved? *International Journal Of Social Psychiatry* 33(4), 312-315.

Wilson H.S. & Kneisel C.R. (1988) *Psychiatric Nursing* 3rd edn. Addison-Wesley, Wokingham.

REFERENCES

BROCKUP, D.Y. and HASTINGS-TOLSMA, M.T. (1995) *Fundamentals Of Research* (2nd ed.), Boston: Jones and Bartlett.

BURNARD, H.R. (1994) *Research Methods in Anthropology: Qualitative and quantitative approaches*, Sage Publications.

BOWERS, L. (1992) Ethnomethodology 1: An Approach To Nursing Research, *International Journal Of Nursing Studies*, 29(1), 59-68.

CLIFFORD, C. and GOUGH, S. (1990) *Nursing Research - A Skills-Based Introduction*, Prentice Hall.

CLIFFORD, C., CARNWELL R. and HARKIN, L. (1997), *Research Methodology in Nursing and Healthcare*, OLF/Churchill Livingstone, Edinburgh.

CLIFFORD, C. and HARKIN, L. (1997) *Inferential Statistics in Nursing and Healthcare*, OLF/Churchill Livingstone, Edinburgh.

CORMACK, D.F.S. (1991) *The Research Process In Nursing* (2nd Ed), Blackwell Scientific Publications.

FIELD, P.A. and MORSE, J. (1996) *Nursing Research: The application of qualitative approaches*, Chapman and Hall.

GLASER, B. and STRAUSS, A. (1967) *The Discovery of Grounded Theory*, Aldine, Chicago.

HAMMERSLEY, M. (1993) *Social Research Philosophy, Politics and Practice*, Sage Publications, London.

KEEBLE, S.(1995) *Experimental Research 1 & 2*, OLF/Churchill Livingstone, Edinburgh.

MILES, M.B. and HUBERMANS, A. M. (1994) *Qualitative Data Analysis*, Sage Publications.

MILLER, H. (1995) *Descriptive Statistics*, OLF/Churchill Livingstone, Edinburgh.

MORGAN, D.L. (1993) 'Qualitative Content Analysis: a guide to paths not taken', *Qualitative Health Research*, Vol. 3, 1., 112-114 February.

MORSE, J.M. (1992) *Qualitative Health Research*, Sage Publications.

MOUSTAKIS, C. (1994) *Phenomenological Research Methods*, Sage Publications.

ROBINSON, K. and VAUGHAN, B. (1992) *Knowledge For Nursing Practice* , Butterworth- Heinemann.

SILVERMAN, D.(1994) *Interpreting Qualitative Data* , Sage Publications.

STRAUSS, A. and CORBIN, J. (1990) *Basics of Qualitative Research*, Sage Publications.

TAYLOR, B. (1994) *Being Human: Ordinariness in Nursing* , Churchill Livingstone, Edinburgh.

GLOSSARY

Analysis –

the process of interpreting **data**.

Anthropological research –

the study of people in institutional and social settings.

Bias –

any unintended influence on research that may distort the findings.

Closed question –

the kind of question in which a researcher expects a limited range of responses. Contrasts with an open question.

Content analysis –

the process of analysing data using words rather than figures.

Convenience sample –

a sample from a **population** selected on the basis of accessibility to the researcher rather than on the basis of **random sample** procedures.

Data –

the information collected in the course of a research study. This may be in numerical form (**quantitative**) or in written or verbal form (**qualitative**).

Data collection techniques –

ways in which **data** or information can be collected, such as a questionnaire, interview, or through observation.

Deductive reasoning –

taking a known idea or theory and applying it to a situation.

Descriptive research –

an approach to research in which the researcher describes what is observed. There is no attempt to control or manipulate **variables**. May be used as a form of **exploratory research**.

Descriptive statistics –

a type of statistics used to describe and summarise data effect. For example, the **data** from a research study may be presented in percentages as a means of summarising large sets of **data**.

Ethnography –

an approach to research influenced by the anthropological tradition, in which the researcher seeks to understand human behaviour from the perspective of the individual in a given culture.

Experimental design –

an approach to research in which the researcher controls the independent variable and measures the effect on the dependent variable in an attempt to look for cause and effect.

Exploratory research –

a term used by researchers beginning to explore a specific phenomenon. Most commonly used with **descriptive research**.

Extraneous variable –

any **variable** other than the **independent variable** which may influence the effect to be measured.

Field notes –

the notes kept by a researcher undertaking an observation study 'in the field', a natural setting rather than a laboratory.

Focus group interview –

an interview technique in which a group of individuals are interviewed simultaneously.

Generalisability –

the extent to which the findings from a study sample can be generalised to the **population** from which the sample was taken.

Grounded theory –

an approach to research in which the aim is to collect and analyse qualitative data in order to develop theory which is 'grounded' in the **data**.

Inductive reasoning –

using **observation** to formulate an idea or theory rather than using known ideas or theories.

Inferential statistics –

a procedure in which statistical tests are used to infer whether the observations in the sample studied are likely to occur in a larger population.

Interview –

an approach used in research in which the researcher collects **data** by face-to-face contact with the subject being studied.

Interview schedule –

the general format used to interview a subject, usually a **questionnaire**.

Literature review –

critical review of the literature relating to an area of research.

Literature search –

the process of finding published literature relating to an area of research.

Observation –

a research method in which a researcher observes subjects in order to gather **data**. Observation research comprises both 'participation' and 'non-participation' research methods. The participant observer observes the subjects from within by becoming a member of the group he or she is researching. The non-participant observer observes the subjects from without by observing the group in his or her role as a researcher.

Open question –

a way of phrasing a question to gather **data** from respondents in a research study. The question requires the respondent to make an individual response. For example, the researcher may ask 'Please tell me what you think about …'. Contrasts with a **closed question**.

Opportunistic sampling –

the researcher selects a sample simply as the opportunity presents itself, using the principles of **purposive/theoretical sampling** to identify the sample.

Phenomenology –

an approach to research which emphasises and seeks to explore the real life experience of an individual.

Population –

the entire set of subjects in a given group that could form the focus of a study. For example, all people who own television sets could be a population (see **sample**).

Positivist research –

a term used to refer to research in the scientific tradition that involves quantification of **data**.

Purposive/theoretical sampling –

a sampling technique used in qualitative research in which the researcher chooses the sample on the basis of known characteristics or experiences.

Qualitative research methods –

research methods which collect and analyse non-numerical **data** through the use of open-ended questionnaires, **interviews**, video recordings and observations.

Quantitative research methods –

research methods which collect **data** which can be summarised numerically. Questionnaire scales, attitude scales, personality tests, physiological measurements and score sheets are examples of this type of research method.

Questionnaire –

a tool for data collection in research. May be highly structured and contain only **closed questions** or have low structure and contain **open questions**. It is not unusual for questionnaires to have a mix of both open and closed question.

Random sample –

an approach to selecting a **sample** which ensures that each member of the **population** being studied has an equal chance of being selected.

Reliability –

the ability of a measurement procedure to produce the same results when used in different places by different researchers. An example of this could be a ruler – this reliably measures length regardless of when, where or who is using it.

Research design –

refers to the overall plan for data collection and **analysis** in a research study.

Research process –

used to describe the actual procedures involved when implementing the **research design**.

Research proposal –

the plan used to establish the framework for the research study.

Research question –

the question set at the beginning of a research project which may be developed to stated aims or a hypothesis (can also be referred to as the research problem).

Sample –

a smaller group or subset of a particular **population** being studied.

Saturation –

the point at which the researcher gathering and analysing qualitative data feels that no new categories are emerging.

Snowball sampling –

arises from **opportunistic sampling.** When a researcher identifies one respondent he or she asks whether the respondent knows any other people who might fit the sampling requirement.

Structured questionnaire –

the type of questionnaire which consists of **closed questions** which give it a high level of structure (contrasts with semi-structured questionnaires which may contain more **open questions**).

Theoretical sampling –

an approach used in sampling in **grounded theory** in which the sampling technique is based on the concepts that have theoretical relevance to the evolving theory.

Time sampling –

an approach to observation research in which the researcher undertakes observation in blocks of time.

Triangulation –

the use of more than one method of collecting or interpreting **data.** For example, using **observation** and **interviews,** or **structured questionnaires** and **interviews.**

Validity –

the extent to which a research tool measures what it is supposed to measure.

Variable –

the term used to describe the characteristics or features of the objects or people in a research study.